SECOND EDITION

PRIMER OF MEDICAL RADIOBIOLOGY

SECOND EDITION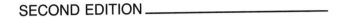

Primer of Medical Radiobiology

Elizabeth LaTorre Travis
Professor, Department of Experimental Radiotherapy
The University of Texas
M. D. Anderson Cancer Center
Houston, Texas

YEAR BOOK MEDICAL PUBLISHERS, INC.
CHICAGO • LONDON • BOCA RATON

1   2   3   4   5   6   7   8   9   0   KR   93   92   91   90   89

Library of Congress Cataloging-in-Publication Data

Travis, Elizabeth LaTorre.
    Primer of medical radiobiology / Elizabeth LaTorre Travis.—2nd
  ed.
        p.   cm.
    Includes bibliographies and index.
    ISBN 0-8151-8837-4
    1. Radiology, Medical.   2. Radiation—Physiological effect.
  I. Title.
    [DNLM: 1. Nuclear Medicine.   2. Radiobiology.   WN 610 T782p]
  R895.T663   1989
  612'.01448—dc19   89-5686
  DNLM/DLC   CIP
  for Library of Congress

Sponsoring Editor: Kevin M. Kelly
Assistant Director, Manuscript Services: Frances M. Perveiler
Production Project Manager: Carol Reynolds
Proofroom Manager: Shirley E. Taylor

To Scott and John

PREFACE TO THE SECOND EDITION

This is the second edition of *Primer of Medical Radiobiology,* which was first published in 1976. Although science is a rapidly expanding area with a constant input of new information, the first edition of this book was not horribly outdated because so much of it dealt with basic concepts and information. However, the time has come to update this textbook, for much has changed in radiobiology in the last 12 years.

This edition, like the former, is intended to provide a basic background in radiation biology to technologists in diagnostic radiology, nuclear medicine, and radiation therapy. Although primarily written with the technologist in mind, the material covered and depth of coverage serve not only those employed in radiation work, e.g., physicists, dosimetrists, and nuclear power plant workers, but also medical students and undergraduate students interested in the effects of radiation on living systems.

This revised edition is organized the same as the first edition, beginning with the effects of radiation at the subcellular and cellular levels and building to the effects on the whole organism in what is hoped is a logical, rational sequence. This edition, like the last, culminates in the medical applications of ionizing radiation. However, this material is now contained in two rather than three chapters (Chapters 9 and 10). This was accomplished by combining diagnostic radiology and nuclear medicine (Chapter 9), since they both use radiation for diagnostic purposes.

Chapters bearing at least some degree of resemblance to their former selves are Chapters 1, 2, 6, and 7—although new, pertinent information has been added to each. For example, Chapter 7, "Total Body Radiation Response," contains the available data from the Russian nuclear power plant accident at Chernobyl.

Chapter 4, "Tissue Radiation Biology," is completely new. Chapters 3 and 10 retain their former titles but contain new, updated information.

Chapters 5, 8, and 9 are updated versions of the originals: Chapter 9 contains the most recent dose estimates for diagnostic procedures, and Chapter 8 contains updated data on the Hiroshima and Nagasaki survivors.

A major technical change in the revised edition is the conversion of dose units to the standard International System of Units (SI units). For example, Gray (Gy) is used instead of rads; it will help the reader to remember that 1 Gy = 100 rads. In some situations it made more sense to use the old dose units, so there are instances where rad, rem, mrem, and similar units are used.

Despite these changes, I have tried not to forget my primary audience and their goals. I have sifted through the last 12-plus years of data and retained that pertinent to technologists. I have attempted to keep this truly a primer and have, hopefully, presented these newer ideas in a clear, readable manner. As in the former edition, concepts and specifics are dealt with, for 12 more years of teaching and researching has reinforced my philosophy that understanding the concept is of fundamental importance to understanding the application.

Elizabeth LaTorre Travis

PREFACE TO THE FIRST EDITION

In recent years the discipline of radiation biology has become a necessary part of medical and allied health school curricula, providing the basis for the many and varied uses of ionizing radiation in the medical profession. As a result, professionals, besides physicians in the three clinical radiology specialties, are expected to and should have a basic knowledge of the biological effects of radiation. This book is intended for just that purpose—to provide a basic background in radiobiology to technologists in diagnostic radiology, nuclear medicine and radiation therapy. Although primarily written with the technologists in mind, the material and depth of coverage should also serve other personnel such as medical and health physicists who are involved in any of the three clinical specialties utilizing ionizing radiation and desire a basic knowledge of biologic events.

Because more and more patients are being referred by an increasing number of physicians to all three radiologic specialties, this book should also be helpful to medical students, residents and physicians in other specialties, providing them the "why's and wherefore's" of the profession. In addition, it can be useful in undergraduate courses in radiation safety, radiobiology and radiation physics.

It cannot be argued that ionizing radiation is a potentially dangerous tool; for this reason, it is imperative that all persons involved with any of the medical applications of ionizing radiation have a basic understanding of its hazardous biologic potential. This knowledge is particularly important in contemporary times as the public is becoming acutely aware of these potential dangers. On the other hand, professionals should not fear this tool, but regard it with a healthy respect. A knowledge of the biologic effects of ionizing radiation will help to promote these attitudes by enhancing the individual's understanding of his chosen profession, thereby enabling him to more effectively function in his field.

I have tried to deal in concepts as well as specifics, with the idea that understanding and knowledge of the basic concepts provides the individual with a greater working knowledge of the topic. Specifics and applications are easily learned if a concept is understood. This book assumes a minimal, not in-depth, knowledge of radiation physics, for the biologic phenomena are a result of physical characteristics of this tool.

Elizabeth LaTorre Travis

ACKNOWLEDGMENTS

No textbook could ever be completed without the assistance of many people. First, I would like to thank all of my colleagues who kindly allowed me to quote their work and reproduce diagrams and illustrations from their own papers. I particularly am grateful to Dr. Eric Hall for his encouragement and generosity in allowing me to quote from his book and papers. The books and papers of Drs. Howard Thames, Rodney Withers, and Jolyon Hendry were also invaluable in the preparation of this text. This book would be much the poorer without their help, as well as the help of many other colleagues, too numerous to mention.

I am grateful to everyone in the art and photography departments at M. D. Anderson Cancer Center, without whose assistance the many superb diagrams in this text would not have been possible. Updating this edition required much library work, and I thank the library staff at M. D. Anderson Cancer Center, particularly Paula Wykoff, for their able assistance.

A special thanks to Leslie Wildrick, Assistant Director, Scientific Publications, who edited the entire manuscript. Her knowledge and skillful use of the English language made for a more readable and understandable text. I am indebted to her for her untiring efforts.

I am deeply indebted to Shelia Buckner, who acted as secretary and editorial assistant. She not only typed the entire manuscript, but edited, collected, and checked material and references and, most importantly, kept me organized. This book would not have been possible without her able assistance.

I am also grateful to the staff in my laboratory who persevered throughout, and to Luka Milas, Chairman of my department, who was encouraging and supportive throughout.

This list would not be complete without mentioning Agnes Potocsny, former Director of the Radiotherapy Technology School at M. D. Anderson Cancer Center, and now our Chief Radiotherapy Technologist, who has been reminding me for 5 years that I really should revise my book.

My thanks also to the technology students, medical students, and residents, who continue to remind me of the responsibilities of a teacher.

And last, but not least, to my family, John, Scott, Debbie, and Pam, for patiently persevering with me.

Elizabeth LaTorre Travis

CONTENTS

Chapter 1 _____

Review of Cell Biology

All living things, whether plants or animals, are made up of organic material called protoplasm. The smallest unit of protoplasm capable of independent existence is the cell. Simple systems may consist of only one cell; however, more complex systems are usually made up of many types of cells, differing in size, shape, and function.

In multicellular systems, cells that serve the same function may be grouped together to form a tissue, e.g., blood and nerve. Some tissues are capable of functioning independently with only one cell type; in most instances, however, several types of tissues exist together to form a functioning unit called an organ, e.g., heart, lungs, and stomach. Organs whose functions are interrelated are then grouped to form systems, such as the cardiovascular, respiratory, and gastrointestinal systems.

Although profound differences exist among the various types of cells in a multicellular organism, certain basic functional and morphologic (structural) characteristics are common to all cells. This chapter reviews these common characteristics and functions of cells.

CHEMICAL COMPOSITION OF THE CELL

Protoplasm consists of inorganic and organic compounds, either dissolved or suspended in water (HOH). Water is the most abundant constituent of protoplasm. In general, protoplasm is 70% to 85% water; but the amount of water varies with cell type. Water serves many functions in the cell and is necessary for life. It is one of the best solvents known; more chemical substances dissolve in water than in most other liquids. Two of the many functions performed by water are as a dispersion medium for compounds in the cell and as a transport vehicle for substances that are utilized by or eliminated from the cell. In addition, most of the physiologic activities that occur in the cell do so largely in water. And, due to its high capacity to absorb and conduct heat, water aids in protecting the cell from drastic temperature changes.

Cell life is virtually impossible without the presence of mineral salts, the inorganic material in the cell. If a cell were placed in water that did not contain salts (i.e., distilled water), it would die. Two examples of salts are sodium (Na) and potassium (K). The concentrations of these salts, K predominantly inside the cell and Na predominantly outside the cell, are vital in ensuring that cell death does not occur from swelling or collapsing. Sodium and potassium perform this function by maintaining the proper proportion of water in the cell (*osmotic pressure*).

Salts also are necessary for the proper functioning of cells and tissues. For example, muscle cramps result from a loss of calcium salts in cells. Salts aid in the production of energy in the cell and in the conduction of impulses along nerves.

There are four major classes of organic compounds in the cell: protein, carbohydrate, nucleic acid, and lipid (Table 1–1). Proteins constitute approximately 15% of cell content and are the most plentiful carbon-containing compounds in the cell. Proteins are composed of simple units joined together to form a long chain complex. These simple units, because they are individually stable and have specific characteristics and properties, are called *monomers*. Structures consisting of monomers joined together to form a chain are termed *polymers*; the process by which polymers are joined is *polymerization*. Another common name for polymers is *macromolecules*; proteins are macromolecules.

The building blocks of a protein are *amino acids*, of which 22 are known in living organisms. These amino acids are linked by a specific type of bond, termed a *peptide bond*. An astounding number of proteins can be derived from the various combinations of these amino acids. A

TABLE 1–1.
Organic Compounds in the Cell

Name	Percent	Components	Examples	Primary Functions
Protein	15	Amino acids	Insulin Albumin Hemoglobin Enzymes	Basic building blocks of cells and tissues
Carbohydrate	1	Carbon Hydrogen Oxygen	Starch Glycogen Lactose Sucrose	Provide energy necessary to all basic cellular functions
Nucleic acid	1	Sugar Phosphate Nitrogenous base	DNA RNA	Direct cellular information and transmit genetic information between cells and generations Role in protein synthesis
Lipid	2	Differs with various types	Cholesterol Castor oil Steroids (vitamin D, sex hormones)	Various functions, e.g., store energy, provide protection

few well-known proteins are insulin, egg white (albumin), gelatin, and hemoglobin.

An important group of proteins in the cell are *enzymes*, a familiar example of which is papain, an ingredient used in commercial meat tenderizer. Enzymes are catalysts, compounds that increase the rate of chemical reactions. The numerous chemical reactions that occur in the cell must do so at very rapid rates; therefore, this group of proteins is essential for the proper functioning of the cell.

Proteins are essential not only to the basic functions of the cell, but also as building blocks of many acellular tissues of the body, such as hair and nails. The importance of this group of organic compounds to all cell life and functions is referred to in the name "protein," from the Greek "prōtos," meaning to occupy first place.

Another class of organic compounds in the cell is carbohydrates, making up approximately 1% of the cell contents. Carbohydrates are composed of carbon, hydrogen, and oxygen, and are the primary source of energy of the cell. This class can be subdivided into three categories: *monosaccharides, disaccharides,* and *polysaccharides.* The first two categories are commonly referred to as sugars, such as table sugar (a disaccharide), and will readily dissolve in water. Polysaccharides are macromolecules, since they consist of a monomer, monosaccharide, polymerized to form a chain.

The third major class of organic compounds, nucleic acid, also may exist as macromolecules in the cell. Two nucleic acids in the cell are deoxyribonucleic acid (*DNA*), and ribonucleic acid (*RNA*). At this point, it is important only to realize that DNA and RNA are polymers; their significance and functions will be discussed in detail later in this chapter.

The final class of organic compounds present in the cell is lipid, more commonly known as fat. Lipids are structural components of the cell membrane and are present in all tissues of the body. This class of organic compounds serves a variety of functions in the cell, such as storage of energy, protection of the body against cold, and assistance in digestive processes.

CELL STRUCTURE

The cell can be divided into two major sections: the *nucleus* and the *cytoplasm*. The nucleus, which is contained within the cytoplasm, is physically separated from it by a membrane, the *nuclear envelope*. This permits the protoplasm of the cell to be accurately described by location as the *nucleoplasm* (within the nucleus) and the *cytoplasm* (outside the nucleus).

When a living cell is examined under the light microscope, its

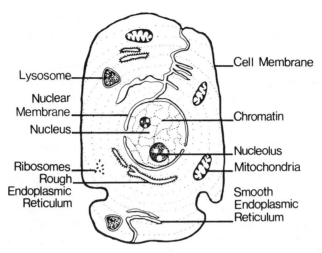

FIG 1–1.
Diagram of the structure of a typical mammalian cell, with representative organelles labeled.

structure is not well defined. With fixation and staining techniques, however, it is possible to visualize more clearly structures in both the nucleus and the cytoplasm; these structures are called *organelles*. Although fixation techniques kill the cell, they do preserve structural integrity; thus, after fixation, the cell retains much of the structural organization present in life. It is also possible to visualize organelles in the cell selectively by using stains that will be absorbed preferentially by certain organelles, thus allowing examination of nuclear and cytoplasmic structures in greater detail.

Cytoplasm

The cytoplasm is the site of all metabolic functions in the cell, including both *anabolism* (building up, *synthesis*) and *catabolism* (breaking down) of organic compounds to provide energy and other requirements for life. Under the light microscope, with the use of staining techniques, the organelles of the cell appear to be suspended in a medium termed the *ground cytoplasm*, or *matrix*. The organelles in the cytoplasm are membrane-limited structures that compartmentalize the cytoplasm. If it were not for these membrane-bound organelles, the cell would not be able to function in the highly organized manner in which it does. Figure 1–1 represents the structure of a typical cell.

Cell Membrane.—Biologists were aware of the existence of a membrane surrounding and encasing the cytoplasm of mammalian cells for many years prior to their ability to examine it (see Fig 1–1). Indirect observations of the functions and structure of this cell membrane produced some early information and theories concerning its structure. Recent technological advances, e.g., the electron microscope and freeze fracture techniques, have made it possible to examine the structure of the cell membrane in greater detail and to determine its constituents; however, the exact configuration remains conjectural. It is known that the cell membrane is predominantly composed of lipids and proteins and appears to be a nonrigid structure.

The main function of the cell membrane is to monitor all exchanges between intracellular (inside the cell) and extracellular (outside the cell) fluid and its contents, thus maintaining the proper physiologic conditions necessary for life. The cell membrane, therefore, is a selectively permeable structure either prohibiting or permitting the passage of substances into and out of the cell. In addition to its permeability, the membrane can conduct an electrical impulse and has a number of enzymatic functions associated with it.

Endoplasmic Reticulum.—Although described in the late 1800s, very little was known about the *endoplasmic reticulum* (ER, or ergastoplasm) until the 1940s when the electron microscope and techniques in high-speed centrifugation became available. The ER, a double-membrane system, is an irregular network of branching and connecting tubules in the cell that has the capability of remodeling itself in response to changes in intracellular physiologic conditions. Because the space between the two membranes of the ER is observed to be continuous with the space between the layers of the nuclear membrane, this organelle is considered to be an extension of the nuclear membrane, and vice versa.

Two types of endoplasmic reticulum have been observed in cells: granular or rough-surfaced ER and smooth or agranular ER (Fig 1–2). Rough ER appears granular when stained due to the presence of ribosomes on its surface. Ribosomes are not present on the surface of agranular ER, giving it a smooth appearance. Thus, the descriptive terminology of "rough" and "smooth" ER is appropriate.

The type of endoplasmic reticulum varies with cell type. In cells that actively synthesize proteins for export, e.g., pancreatic cells that produce insulin, there is an abundance of granular ER. A reduced amount of granular ER is present in cells that are synthesizing proteins predominantly for their own use. However, agranular ER is present in cells that are synthesizing products other than proteins. It is well known that granular ER is involved in protein synthesis, but the role of agranular ER is not entirely known—it seems to have a variety of functions, depending on cell type.

Ribosomes.—Ribosomes are cytoplasmic organelles made up of protein and RNA in approximately equal quantities, either free in the cytoplasm or attached to the endoplasmic reticulum. From the previous discussion of ER, we know that ER with attached ribosomes is actively engaged in protein synthesis; the actual site of protein synthesis in the cell is on the ribosome (see Fig 1–2).

The synthesis of protein by the cell is a highly organized and efficient procedure involving RNA. Essentially, the process is one in which the nucleus, which controls protein synthesis, sends a message to the cytoplasm indicating which protein is to be made. This message,

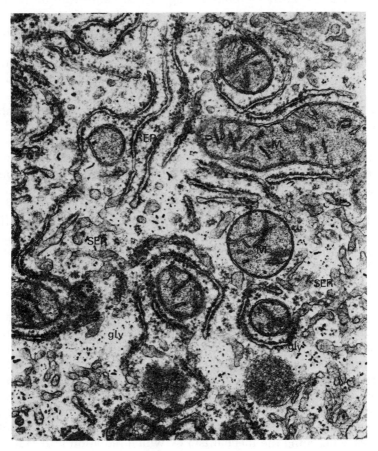

FIG 1–2.
Electron micrograph of the cytoplasm of a normal rat hepatocyte (liver cell) demonstrating *RER*, rough endoplasmic reticulum; *SER*, smooth endoplasmic reticulum; *M*, mitochondria; and *gly*, glycogen. (Magnification × 37,500.)

in the form of a code, is carried by a specific type of RNA appropriately termed "messenger" RNA. The messenger RNA travels to the ribosome, which "reads" the message, translates it, and assembles the amino acids in their proper sequence to form the specific protein. At the end of the process, the protein is released from the ribosome. An interesting fact about this organelle is that, regardless of the biologic system studied, ribosomes are similar in size, shape, and structure.

Mitochondria.—These organelles can be visualized with a light microscope and were first observed in the cell as early as 1890. However, it was not until methods of high-speed centrifugation became available that it was possible to harvest mitochondria in bulk and further examine their structure. Mitochondria are the powerhouses of the cell, producing energy for cellular functions by breaking down (catabolizing) nutrients through a process called oxidation. The major source of energy for the cell is carbohydrate, but lipids also can be used for energy production if necessary.

Mitochondria are elliptical structures limited by a double membrane surrounding a central cavity. The inner membrane is folded inward into the central cavity to form a series of shelflike structures called *cristae* (see Fig 1–2). The specific enzymes necessary for the production of energy are located on the cristae. These enzymes are not randomly distributed in the mitochondria, but are highly organized to facilitate the sequence of catabolic reactions for the production of energy.

The number of mitochondria in any particular cell tends to reflect the energy requirements of that cell. For example, cardiac muscle cells requiring a great deal of energy have a large number of mitochondria; lymphocytes with low energy requirements, on the other hand, have only a few mitochondria.

Lysosomes.—These organelles, first recognized in 1955 as separate entities in the cell, are single-membrane limited structures that contain enzymes capable of breaking down proteins, DNA, and some carbohydrates. These lysosomal enzymes are capable of digesting, or *lysing*, the cell if they are released. Under normal conditions, the enzymes are safely confined within the sac of the lysosome. However, many agents are capable of altering the permeability of the lysosomal membrane, causing release of the enzymes. In fact, this was one of the initial theories concerning the mechanism by which radiation kills cells.

Golgi Complex.—The Golgi complex may exist in a number of morphologic varieties, the most common of which is a stacked set of

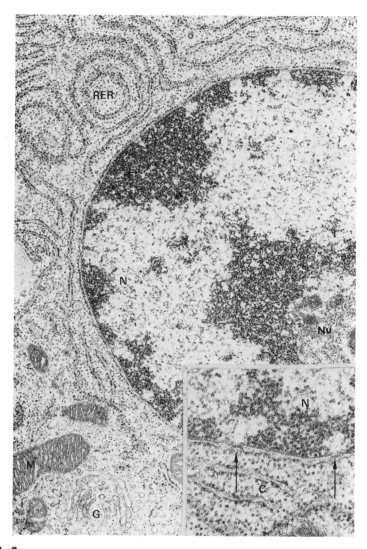

FIG 1–3.
Electron micrograph of a portion of a nucleus and the cytoplasm of a cell from a rat parotid gland: *N*, nucleus; *Nu*, nucleolus; *RER*, rough endoplasmic reticulum; *G*, golgi; *M*, mitochondria. (Magnification × 25,000.) Note the double membrane surrounding the nucleus except in the region of the pores where it is single *(arrows).* (Magnification × 45,000.) (Courtesy of Dr JV Simson.)

double-membrane structures and small vesicles (little spheres) enclosing a space that may be continuous with the space between the membranes of the endoplasmic reticulum (Fig 1–3). Although all of the functions of the Golgi complex have not been defined, experimental evidence suggests that this organelle is involved in a variety of functions including secretion, as a packaging area for products manufactured by the cell for export, carbohydrate synthesis, and the binding of other organic compounds to proteins.

Nucleus

The nucleus, which is contained within the cytoplasm, is physically separated from it by a membrane, the *nuclear envelope*. This is a double membrane, the space between the two membranes being continuous with the space between the membranes of the endoplasmic reticulum. The two membranes of the nuclear envelope fuse at various points to form "pores," which are normally closed by a diaphragm appearing to consist of a dense material (see Fig 1–3). This diaphragm impedes the free exchange of materials between the nucleus and the cytoplasm; however, selective passage of some molecules from the nucleus to the cytoplasm is permitted, as in the case of nuclear RNA. Much of the RNA in the nucleus is contained within a rounded body called the *nucleolus*, which, in some cells, is attached to the nuclear membrane (see Fig 1–3).

Although the nucleus and the cytoplasm are physically separate, they are mutually dependent upon each other for life. Functionally, the cytoplasm is the site of metabolism, but the nucleus supervises and coordinates cytoplasmic activities. Changes in the nucleus can impair its ability to direct cytoplasmic functions; changes in the cytoplasm will affect the nucleus, since the various functions of the cytoplasm keep the nucleus alive and enable it to reproduce and repair itself.

Table 1–2 summarizes the location and function of cellular organelles.

DNA.—Contained within the nucleus is the DNA molecule which, in code form, contains genetic information. DNA is a double-stranded structure twisted upon itself to form a tightly coiled molecule resembling a spiral staircase. This configuration is termed a *double helix* (Fig 1–4). The name "deoxyribonucleic acid" indicates the units that make up this macromolecule. The subunits of DNA are a nitrogenous base, a 5-carbon sugar, and phosphoric acid. These three components taken together are called a *nucleotide* or, in this case, deoxyribose nucleotide (Table 1–3).

If we unwind the DNA macromolecule and consider it as a ladder, we see that the side rails of the ladder (the "backbone" of DNA) are composed of sugar molecules joined by a common phosphoric acid

TABLE 1–2.

Cellular Organelles

Name	Location	Function
Cell membrane	Cytoplasm	Monitors exchanges between cell and environment
Endoplasmic reticulum	Cytoplasm	
Rough ER		Protein synthesis
Smooth ER		Variety of functions in cells, making substances other than protein
Ribosomes	Cytoplasm	Protein synthesis
Mitochondria	Cytoplasm	Produce energy by oxidizing carbohydrates and lipids
Lysosomes	Cytoplasm	Contains enzymes capable of destroying the cell
Golgi complex	Cytoplasm	Concentration and segregation of products for secretion; carbohydrate synthesis
Nuclear membrane	Nucleus	Separation of nucleus from cytoplasm; permits selective passage of molecules from nucleus to cytoplasm, and vice versa
Nucleolus	Nucleus	Contains RNA
Nucleus	DNA	Contains genetic information

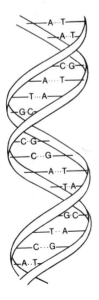

FIG 1–4.
Double helical structure of DNA and the relationship of the four bases to the backbone. *A,* adenine; *T,* thymine; *G,* guanine; *C,* cytosine.

TABLE 1–3.

Chemical
Composition of
DNA

Nucleotide
Phosphoric acid
Sugar
Base

TABLE 1–4.

Bases in DNA

Purines	Pyrimidines
Adenine (A)	Thymine (T)
Guanine (G)	Cytosine (C)

molecule (a *phosphate bond*). The rungs of the ladder are made up of the nitrogenous bases (Fig 1–5). These bases are important constituents of DNA because they are the only units that differ in the macromolecule. The sugar and the phosphoric acid are the same along the DNA strand; however, there are only four kinds of nitrogenous bases present in DNA. These four bases are divided into two categories: the purines, which are adenine and guanine, and the pyrimidines, which are thymine and cytosine (Table 1–4). A base is bonded to a sugar molecule on one or the other side of the ladder. The bases then join the two side rails of the DNA ladder by pairing with each other through hydrogen bonds.

These bases, the purines and the pyrimidines, do not bond randomly with each other, but can pair only in a very specific manner. A purine pairs only with a pyrimidine—purines and pyrimidines never pair with themselves. What is even more fascinating in view of DNA's

FIG 1–5.
Ladderlike configuration of an unspiraled DNA molecule. Sugar molecules joined by phosphate (PO_4) bonds *(solid line)* form the side rails; nitrogenous bases bonded to each other *(broken line)* and to a sugar molecule on each side rail *(solid line)* form the rungs joining the two backbones.

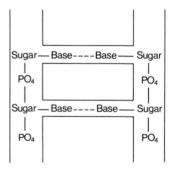

major role in cell life is that one specific purine can only pair with one specific pyrimidine, i.e., adenine pairs only with thymine and guanine pairs only with cytosine. Because of this characteristic, the two strands of DNA are said to be complementary to each other.

DNA is ultimately responsible for directing cellular activity and for transmitting genetic information from cell to cell and from generation to generation. The order that exists in the cell is due to the unique component of the DNA molecule, the nitrogenous base. Because of the uniqueness and specific pairing of the nitrogenous bases, these remarkable constituents determine the genetic information available to the cell, not by themselves, but by their linear sequence on the DNA molecule.

This is an astounding concept, considering that the various arrangements of only four molecules provide much of the diversity in life as we know it. Even more astonishing is the effect that a single change in one of the bases or in their linear sequence can have on a cell. This alteration of the information carried by DNA, termed a mutation, may be so slight that it will not be grossly manifested by the cell, or it may be a major alteration resulting in cell death. Because of the profound impact any change in DNA can have on the cell, DNA is considered the likely candidate for the primary target of radiation-induced cell death.

DNA, Genes, and Chromosomes.—In the nucleus, DNA is contained within long thread-like structures called chromosomes, a word derived from Latin meaning "colored bodies." Chromosomes, visible only in dividing cells, appear as dark-stained linear bodies which are constricted at certain points by a structure called the *centromere*, a clear region necessary to the movement of the chromosome during cell division. The extensions of the chromosome on either side of the centromere are termed "arms." The structure of a typical chromosome is given in Figure 1–6.

Arranged on each chromosome are genes, each of which contains a finite segment of DNA with a specific base sequence. One chromosome contains many genes arranged in a specific linear sequence. The human genome contains about 60,000 genes with 2×10^9 bases. The genes are units of genetic material responsible for directing cytoplasmic activity and transmitting hereditary information in the cell. A schematic diagram of the relationship between chromosomes, genes, and DNA is shown in Figure 1–6.

In general, there are two types of cells in sexually reproducing plants and animals, germ cells (*gametes*: female—oocytes;

male—spermatozoa) and *somatic* cells (all other cells). These two types of cells differ in the amount of genetic material they contain. In each somatic cell, there are at least two of each kind of gene located on two different chromosomes. These two chromosomes are alike in the sequence and type of genes they carry, and are called *homologues.* Therefore, in somatic cells, the chromosomes are paired; each member of a pair is alike, but the pairs are all different.

The number of chromosomes in somatic cells is referred to as the *diploid* or 2n number, which is constant for a given species of plant or animal. However, the 2n number of chromosomes varies with different species; e.g., in humans 2n equals 46, in dogs 2n equals 78, in cats 2n equals 38, and in gorillas and chimpanzees 2n equals 48.

In germ cells, chromosomes are not paired but exist singly. These individual chromosomes are one of the homologous chromosomes from each of the pairs present in somatic cells. Therefore, the number of

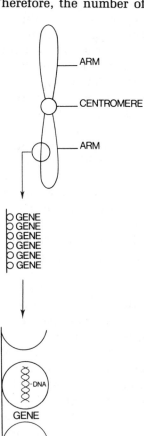

FIG 1–6.
Relationship of a chromosome, genes, and DNA. **Top,** structure of a typical chromosome. Although shown in the center, the centromere is not located at this site on all chromosomes. **Middle,** enlarged area of the chromosome demonstrating the relationship of genes on the chromosome. **Bottom,** enlargement of one gene, relating DNA to the gene.

chromosomes and genes in germ cells is one half the number found in somatic cells. This specific number of chromosomes in germ cells is called the n or *haploid* number.

Although most somatic cells would die or function abnormally with less than the 2n number of chromosomes, germ cells can exist with only one half this number due to their specialization. Metabolically, the germ cells do not require or perform all of the functions of somatic cells; therefore, their limited metabolism makes survival possible with less than the full complement of chromosomes.

Functionally, the germ cells have one specific purpose—they are responsible for reproduction of the species. During fertilization, the male and female gametes unite to form the zygote (fertilized egg). Therefore, by necessity, each germ cell must contain only one half the number of chromosomes to produce a normal zygote containing the essential 2n number of chromosomes.

CELL DIVISION AND THE CELL CYCLE

Somatic Cells

During fetal development and growth, a majority (if not all) of the cells of the body are dividing. In adult life, tissues neither grow nor shrink, although some of them contain actively dividing cells. In this latter situation, then, cell production must be balanced by cell loss, i.e., a steady state exists. In somatic cells, the process by which mammalian cells proliferate is termed *mitosis*. In this process one parent cell divides and forms two identical daughter cells, resulting in an equal (approximately) distribution of all cellular materials between the two daughter cells—two cells that are exact copies of the parent cell.

Mitosis

Mitosis itself can be divided into four phases: prophase, metaphase, anaphase, and telophase.

Prophase.—In early prophase, the genetic material initially appears granular, gradually forming delicate, elongated strands evenly distributed throughout the nucleus (Fig 1–7,A). These delicate strands are the first signs of chromosomal formation. As prophase progresses, the two chromatids of each chromosome shorten and thicken and can be observed moving toward the intact nuclear envelope. During late prophase the nuclear membrane begins to break down, leaving a clear zone in

FIG 1–7.
Mitosis in a somatic cell containing four sister chromatids. **A,** prophase—chromatin becomes filamentous and visible. **B,** metaphase—chromatids aligned on the equatorial plate. **C,** anaphase—migration of chromatids along spindle to opposite poles of the cell. **D,** telophase, reconstruction of the nuclear membrane and cytokinesis complete the mitotic process.

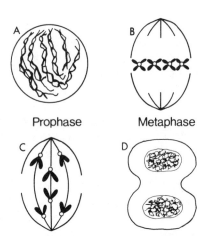

Prophase   Metaphase

Anaphase   Telophase

the center of the cell. The chromosomes now move randomly in this zone as they approach the center of the cell (the *equatorial plate*). This signals the initiation of the second phase of mitosis, metaphase. One other important event occurs during prophase, the formation of the *spindle.* The spindle is made up of delicate fibers that extend from one side (pole) of the cell to the other. These fibers are attached at opposite poles of the cell to structures called *centrioles.*

Metaphase.—Metaphase begins when the chromosomes line up in the center of the cell, forming the equatorial plate (Fig 1–7,B). The nuclear membrane is completely broken down at this time, and the chromosomes are free to move around in the cell. The two chromatids of each chromosome now attach to the spindle by means of the centromere, and begin to repel each other with their "arms" pointed toward the center of the cell and the centromere pointed toward the pole. Until metaphase, the two chromatids of each chromosome share a common centromere. During metaphase, however, the centromere is duplicated, allowing each chromatid to individually attach to the spindle. The migration of the chromatids along the spindle signals the initiation of anaphase.

Anaphase.—During anaphase, the two chromatids repel each other and migrate along the spindle to opposite poles of the cell (Fig 1–7,C). At the completion of anaphase, each duplicated chromosome is located at opposite poles of the cell; this marks the beginning of the last phase of mitosis.

Telophase.—During telophase, the chromosomes lose their definitive appearance and become elongated strands, eventually assuming a homogenous appearance in the nucleus. Simultaneously, the nuclear membrane is reconstructed around the genetic material (Fig 1–7,D). In essence, telophase is the reverse process of prophase.

In addition to nuclear reconstruction, division of the cytoplasm (*cytokinesis*) also occurs during telophase. Indentation of the cell membrane begins to divide the cytoplasm in the vicinity of the equator of the cell. By this process the cytoplasm is divided approximately equally between the two daughter cells. Cytokinesis continues until the cytoplasm is completely separated, forming two daughter cells, each having a complete cell membrane.

At the end of telophase the two daughter cells formed are comparable to the original parent cell and contain a full complement of chromosomes (2n set). The cell has now completed mitosis. Essentially, the process of mitosis maintains genetic continuity and preserves the status quo. Figure 1–8 shows photomicrographs of the various stages of mitosis of human cells in tissue culture.

For many years, only these four phases of mitosis could be observed under the light microscope. At the same time, it was also observed that most cells were not dividing but were between successive mitoses in a "resting" phase, termed *interphase*.

Interphase.—Microscopically, the interphase nucleus appears nondescript (Fig 1–9). When the DNA is stained, the genetic material appears clumped in different patterns throughout the nucleoplasm, depending on cell type and function. Individual chromosomes are *not* visible during interphase. Due to this microscopic appearance, interphase was referred to for many years as the "resting" phase of cell division. Improved biochemical techniques and increased use of radionuclides allowed indirect observation and measurement of the cell's activities during interphase, quickly dispelling the idea that this phase is a nondynamic resting period.

As previously stated, somatic cells contain the diploid number of chromosomes and divide by the process of mitosis, defined as the division of nuclear and cytoplasmic material between two daughter cells, maintaining the integrity of life of the parent cell. The daughter cells must have not only the diploid number of chromosomes, but also the same genes and, therefore, an identical sequence of bases on the DNA molecule as the parent cell. At some point in the cell cycle prior to mitosis, DNA must be duplicated (synthesized) and its integrity maintained. The first light shed on the activities of the cell during interphase was by Howard and Pelc in 1952, who found that DNA was synthesized during at least a portion of interphase.

DNA Synthesis.—The process of DNA synthesis doubles the amount of original DNA in such a manner that the new DNA molecules are

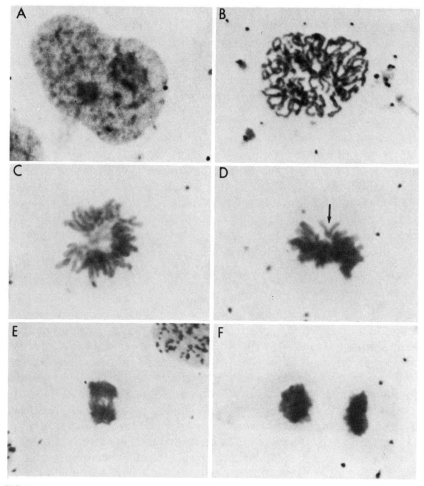

FIG 1–8.
Photomicrograph of mitosis in a human epithelial cell (HeLa) grown in tissue culture; only the chromosomes are stained. **A,** interphase. **B,** early prophase, note filamentous structure of chromatin. **C,** late prophase, chromosomes approaching equatorial plate. **D,** metaphase chromosomes line up, forming equatorial plate in a classic view of metaphase. Note visible centromere and arms of one chromosome *(arrow)*. **E,** anaphase, chromosomes pulling apart, approaching opposite poles of the cell. **F,** telophase, chromosomes lose their distinct appearance as the cell approaches interphase. (Feulgen stain, magnification × 2,000.)

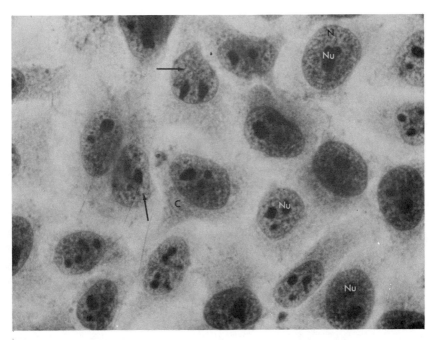

FIG 1–9.
Photomicrograph of human cervical carcinoma cells illustrating the nucleus *(N)* with visible chromatin *(arrows)*, nucleolus *(Nu)*, and cytoplasm *(C)*. Cytoplasmic organelles cannot be seen. (H & E stain, magnification × 1,000.)

identical to the original molecule. The two strands of the original molecule each act as a mold or template upon which a new complementary strand of DNA is synthesized. Initially, the DNA molecule unwinds from its double helical, ladderlike configuration; the bond between two of the bases forming the rungs of the ladder is broken, and the two side rails (backbone) of the DNA ladder separate, leaving an unpaired purine and pyrimidine base on each strand of the original molecule. Within the cell there is a storehouse of "new" purine and pyrimidine bases, which will correctly pair with the unpaired purine and pyrimidine on the two chains of the original DNA molecule. For example, if adenine was on one of the original chains, only thymine will pair with it. On the opposite chain of the original molecule, only a new adenine will bond with the unpaired thymine. A new backbone of sugar and phosphate is simultaneously constructed, thus completing a section of the new chain.

This process continues gradually along each strand of the original DNA molecule until two completely new strands of DNA have been synthesized that are complementary to the original strands (Fig 1–10).

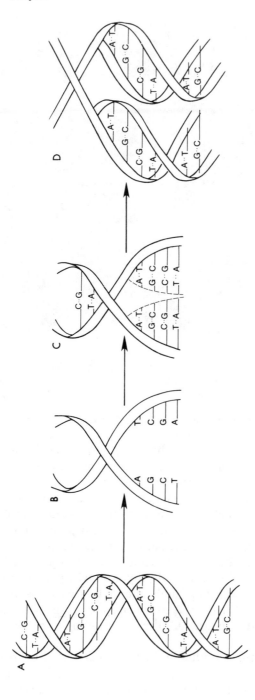

FIG 1–10.

Schematic of DNA replication. **A,** DNA before replication. Note base sequence on molecule. **B,** unwinding and separation of portion of the DNA molecule signals the initiation of DNA replication. Note the unpaired bases on each strand of the molecule. **C,** a storehouse of bases in the cell provides the appropriate partner to join with the unpaired bases on each chain (*dotted lines* indicate site of new backbone). **D,** new backbones are constructed, producing two complete DNA molecules—*both* molecules identical in base composition to the parent. This process continues along the DNA chain until the whole molecule is replicated. *A,* adenine; *T,* thymine; *C,* cytosine; *G,* guanine.

The net result is two DNA molecules that are exact copies (replicas) of the original, providing the necessary complement of DNA to form two daughter cells during mitosis. Therefore, the process of DNA synthesis is often termed *replication* and is designated "**S.**"

It has been found that the process of DNA synthesis does not involve all of interphase. Between telophase and the beginning of DNA synthesis, there is a period called "**G_1,**" (G designating "gap"), when DNA is not replicating. After DNA has been synthesized, there is another period before the cell begins mitosis when DNA is not replicating; this period is termed "**G_2.**" At the end of G_2 the cell enters the first phase of mitosis, prophase.

This cyclic process is referred to as the cell cycle, and is diagrammed in Figure 1–11. A fifth phase, **G_0,** has been added to the cell cycle to account for cells that show no evidence of progressing through division for very long periods. Although these cells are not committed to divide as cells in other phases of the cycle are, they retain their capability to divide and can be recruited into the cell cycle and mitosis, if necessary. These cells, which may represent true "resting" cells, are often termed quiescent (**Q**) cells.

Many techniques now permit an estimation of the length of the various phases of the cell cycle. All of them rely on selective visualization of dividing cells, either by the human eye or by an instrument called the flow cytometer. Both techniques require a method of staining the DNA in the cells to make it visible either to the human eye or to the laser beam of the flow cytometer. In the original work of Howard and Pelc, the DNA precursor thymidine (which would be incorporated only in dividing cells) was tagged with a radioactive label, tritium. Using autoradiography, the cells in DNA synthesis at the time the label

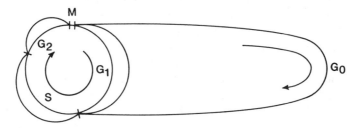

FIG 1–11.
Diagram of the cell cycle showing that the time of mitosis is relatively constant, whereas the most variable phase is G_1. The G_0 period has been postulated for cells that usually do not divide but are capable of being recruited into the cell cycle and division, if necessary. For example, liver cells normally do not divide, but after removal of part of the liver (partial hepatectomy), these cells can and do divide. Such cells are termed quiescent cells.

was present could be visualized by light microscopy and manually counted, allowing the lengths of the phases of the cycle to be estimated. Although tedious, this technique provides useful information. However, these same parameters can be more easily and rapidly estimated using the newly developed method of flow cytometry, which employs a laser beam to quantitate the fluorescence of cells stained with a fluorescent dye.

Both methods have shown that there is a large variation in the cell cycle time (i.e., the time from the beginning of one mitosis to the beginning of the next by the daughter cells). However, there is a surprising consistency in the times different cells spend in some phases of the cycle. Mitosis, once it begins, lasts only about 1 hour in all cells. The S period, the time of DNA synthesis, is also remarkably uniform and takes no longer than 15 hours. The G_2 period occupies about 1 to 5 hours of the entire cycle. The differences, then, between the cell cycle times of various cells can be accounted for by a dramatic variation in the length of the G_1 period.

GERM CELLS

Meiosis

Meiosis is the process by which germ cells divide. This is a specialized type of cell division that reduces the number of chromosomes in the oocyte and spermatozoan from the diploid number (2n) to the haploid number (n). As previously stated, a reduction in the chromosome number of germ cells is necessary if the zygote is to contain the diploid number. If the chromosomes of the germ cells were not reduced from 2n to n (in humans, from 46 to 23), the zygote would receive twice the essential number of chromosomes.

Meiosis is a process of reduction division in which the cell divides twice in succession but the chromosomes are duplicated only once. In germ cells, as in somatic cells, DNA synthesis occurs during interphase, and the net result is the same—DNA replicates, resulting in a duplication of each chromosome, forming two chromatids. Therefore, the germ cell begins meiosis with double the amount of genetic material.

The names for the phases of meiosis and mitosis are the same. During meiosis, the movements of germ cell chromosomes are very similar to the movements of somatic cell chromosomes during mitosis. At the end of telophase, the original parent germ cell has formed two daughter cells with 2n number of chromosomes. However, the similarities between mitosis and meiosis end at this point.

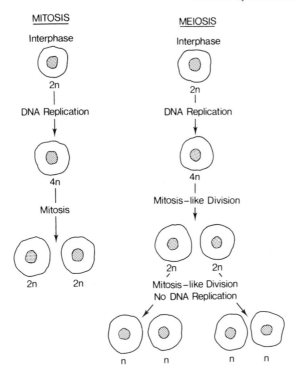

FIG 1–12.
Comparing mitosis and meiosis. **Left,** mitosis. Process of division in somatic cells. One parent cell with 2*n* chromosomes forms two daughter cells, each with 2*n* chromosomes, thus maintaining the status quo. Note only one DNA replication process and one division of the cell occurs during mitosis. **Right,** meiosis. One parent germ cell with 2*n* chromosomes forms four daughter cells, each with *n* chromosomes. Note the first process of meiosis is the same as mitosis, producing two daughter cells with 2*n* chromosomes; at this point the major difference occurs: germ cells divide again without DNA replication, producing four daughter cells, each with *n* chromosomes.

These daughter cells now undergo a second division of all cellular material, including the chromosomes, without replication of DNA and thus without duplication of the chromosomes. The consequence of these two successive divisions of meiosis is four gametes, each containing the haploid number of chromosomes. A diagrammatic comparison of the processes of mitosis and meiosis is given in Figure 1–12.

One other important event occurs during meiosis, termed "crossing over." In essence, *crossing over* is the exchange of genes between sister chromatids, allowing for increased genetic variability within a species.

REFERENCES

1. Bloom W, Fawcett DW: *A Textbook of Histology*, ed 9. Philadelphia, WB Saunders, 1969.
2. Bresnick E, Schwartz A: *Functional Dynamics of the Cell*. New York, Academic Press, 1968.
3. Davidson JN: *Biochemistry of Nucleic Acids*, ed 5. London, Methuen & Co, 1965.
4. DeRobertis ED, et al: *Cell Biology*, ed 5. Philadelphia, WB Saunders, 1970.
5. Gray JW, Dolbeare F, Pallavicini MG, et al: Cell cycle analysis using flow cytometry. *Int J Radiat Biol* 1986; 49:237–255.
6. Howard H, Pelc SR: Synthesis of deoxyribonucleic acid in normal and irradiated cells and its relation to chromosome breakage. *Heredity (Suppl)* 1952; 6:261.
7. Koehler JK: *Biological Electron Microscopy*. Berlin, Springer-Verlag, 1973.
8. Watson JD: *Molecular Biology of the Gene*. New York, WA Benjamin, 1965.
9. White A, et al: *Principles of Biochemistry*, ed 4. New York, McGraw-Hill Book Co, 1968.

Chapter 2 _____

Basic Biologic Interactions of Radiation

_____

The biologic effects of ionizing radiation represent the efforts of living things to deal with energy absorbed by them after an interaction with such radiation. Radiobiology is the study of the sequence of events that follows the absorption of energy from ionizing radiation, the efforts of the organism to compensate for the effects of this energy absorption, and the damage to the organism that may be produced.

When discussing the changes that occur in biologic material after an interaction with ionizing radiation, the following generalizations are important to keep in mind:

1. The interaction of radiation in cells is a probability function or a matter of chance, i.e., it may or may not interact and, if interaction occurs, damage may or may not be produced.
2. The initial deposition of energy occurs very rapidly—in a period of approximately 10^{-17} second.
3. Radiation interaction in a cell is nonselective. The energy from ionizing radiation is deposited randomly in the cell; no areas of the cell are "chosen" by the radiation.
4. The visible changes in the cells, tissues, and organs resulting from an interaction with ionizing radiation are not unique—they cannot be distinguished from damage produced by other types of trauma.
5. The biologic changes in cells and tissues resulting from radiation occur only after a period of time (*latent period*), the length of which depends on the initial dose and varies from minutes to weeks, or even years.

BASIC INTERACTIONS OF RADIATION

Understanding the visible response of cells, tissues, and organisms to ionizing radiation requires an understanding of the initial interactions of radiation in the cell. Extensive research has defined the initial changes that lead to the visible response of the cell, tissue, or organism.

When ionizing radiation interacts with a cell, ionizations and excitations* are produced either in critical biologic macromolecules called targets (e.g., DNA) or in the medium in which the cellular organelles are suspended (e.g., water, HOH). Based on the site of these interactions, the action of radiation on the cell can be classified as either direct or indirect.

Direct action is well described by its name: it occurs when any type of radiation deposits its energy directly in the critical target, resulting

---

*Excitation is a result of radiation interaction in the cell, a possible consequence of which is damage. Once believed to be relatively inefficient for causing damage in molecules, excitation has been shown to have a high efficiency for causing bond breakage, and therefore damage, in some systems. In general, the effects of excitation on a molecule vary with the complexity and inherent stability of the molecule. The reader should refer to a text on basic radiation physics for further discussion of this phenomenon.

in ionization or excitation of this target. Thus, the chain of events that eventually leads to biologic damage has begun. Although it was stated above that direct action can occur with any type of radiation, it is more likely to occur after exposure to high-LET (linear energy transfer) radiations, such as particles or neutrons, than after exposure to sparsely ionizing radiation, such as x-rays. In fact, direct action is the dominant process whereby damage occurs after high-LET radiations. (This will be discussed in the next chapter.) Direct action, then, produces damage by direct ionization of the critical target.

Indirect action also is an appropriate descriptive term, for, in this type of damage, the critical site is damaged by reactive species produced by ionizations elsewhere in the cell, which in turn damage the target. Since 80% of the cell consists of water, indirect action primarily occurs through ionization of water molecules.

If the products of the interaction of radiation with water are responsible for damage to the target, first they must be able to diffuse far enough to reach the target, and second, they must be in a form that will damage it. Such highly reactive diffusible species are produced when radiation interacts with water, and are termed free radicals. Free radicals, symbolized by a dot (e.g., OH˙ or H˙), contain a single unpaired electron in their outer shells, a state which renders them chemically unstable. The chemical stability of an atom or molecule is due to its having an even number of electrons that also are paired in spin; i.e., for each electron spinning clockwise, another spins in the counterclockwise direction. Free radicals have an uneven number of electrons that also are not paired in spin, a state which confers a high degree of reactivity.

Basically, the absorption of radiation by a water molecule results in the production of an ion pair (HOH^+, HOH^-). This occurs through the following reaction:

$$HOH \xrightarrow{\text{Radiation}} HOH^+ + e^-$$

The free electron (e^-) is captured by another water molecule, forming the second ion:

$$HOH + e^- \rightarrow HOH^-$$

The two ions produced by the above reactions are unstable and rapidly dissociate (break down), provided normal water molecules are present, forming another ion and a free radical by the following reactions:

$$HOH^+ \rightarrow H^+ + OH^{\cdot}*$$

$$HOH^- \rightarrow OH^- + H^{\cdot}$$

The ultimate result of the interaction of radiation with water is the formation of an ion pair (H^+, OH^-) and free radicals ($H^{\cdot}$, $OH^{\cdot}$). The consequences of these products to the cell are many and varied. The ion pair may react in one of two ways:

1. They may recombine and form a normal water molecule ($H^+ + OH^- = HOH$). The net effect in this case will be no damage to the cell.
2. They may chemically react and damage cellular macromolecules.

Generally, because the H^+ and OH^- ions do not contain excessive amounts of energy, the probability that they will recombine without causing damage in the cell is great, provided they are in the vicinity of each other.

The free radicals that result from the above reactions are extremely reactive due to their chemical and physical properties, and can undergo a number of reactions, a few of which are:

1. Recombining with each other producing no damage, e.g., $H^{\cdot} + OH^{\cdot} \rightarrow H_2O$.
2. Joining with other free radicals, possibly forming a new molecule that may be damaging to the cell, e.g., $OH^{\cdot} + OH^{\cdot} \rightarrow H_2O_2$ (hydrogen peroxide, an agent toxic to the cell).
3. Reacting with normal molecules and biologic macromolecules in the cell, forming new or damaged structures, e.g., $H^{\cdot} + O_2 \rightarrow HO_2$ (free radical combined with oxygen forming a new free radical); $RH + H^{\cdot} \rightarrow R^{\cdot} + H_2$ (free radical reacts with a biologic molecule [RH], removing H and forming a biologic free radical).

The effects of free radicals in the cell are compounded by their ability to initiate chemical reactions—and, therefore, damage—at distant sites in the cell. Although many other reactions occur and many other products are formed by the interaction of radiation with water, free radicals, particularly the OH radical, are believed to be a major factor in the production of damage via indirect action in the cell.

---

*Experimental data suggest that about two thirds of all damage in the cell that occurs via indirect action is caused by the highly reactive OH radical.

The following outline summarizes the general sequence of events that occurs in the cell via indirect action.[†]

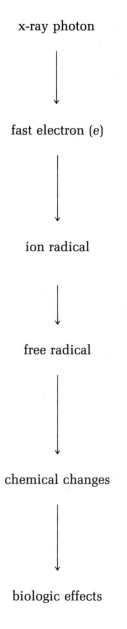

x-ray photon

fast electron (e)

ion radical

free radical

chemical changes

biologic effects

[†]Adapted from Hall EJ: *Radiobiology for the Radiologist*, ed 3. Philadelphia, JB Lippincott, 1988.

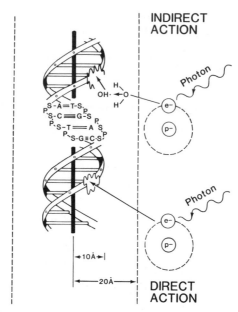

FIG 2–1.
Schematic of the direct and indirect actions of radiation on DNA. The letters *S* and *P* represent the sugar and phosphate backbone of the DNA molecule, and *A, T, C,* and *G* represent the four bases adenine, thymine, guanine, and cytosine. In direct action, an ejected electron produced by the absorption of radiation interacts directly with the DNA molecule, whereas in indirect action the ejected electron interacts with a water molecule, producing free radicals, which in turn damage the DNA molecule. (Redrawn from Hall EJ: *Radiobiology for the Radiologist,* ed 3. Philadelphia, JB Lippincott, 1988, p 11. Used by permission.)

It is important to keep in mind that because there is more water in the cell than any other structural component, the probability of radiation damage occurring through indirect action is much greater than the probability of damage occurring through direct action. In addition, indirect action occurs *primarily* but not *exclusively* from free radicals that result from the ionization of water. The ionization of other cellular constituents, particularly fat, also can result in free radical formation.

In summary, *direct action* produces damage by direct ionization of a biologic macromolecule; *indirect action* produces damage through chemical reactions initiated by the ionization of water. In both cases the primary interaction (ionization) is the same; the definition of direct and indirect action depends on the *site* of ionization and energy absorption in the cell. Figure 2–1 presents a comparison of direct and indirect action in the cell.

TABLE 2–1.

LET Values

Type of Radiation	LET (keV/μm)
Cobalt 60	0.3
3 meV x-ray	0.3
250 keV x-ray	3.0
5 meV α-particle	100.0
Neutron	
19.0 meV	7.0
2.5 meV	20.0
Electron	
1.0 meV	0.25
1.0 keV	12.3

LET AND RBE

Linear energy transfer (LET) is the rate at which energy is deposited as a charged particle travels through matter by a particular type of radiation. Expressed in keV/μm, or energy deposited per unit distance of path traveled by the particle, LET is a function of the mass and charge of the radiation. Electromagnetic radiation (x- and γ-rays), although having no mass or charge, produces fast electrons—particles with negligible mass and a charge of -1. Because of these physical properties, the probability of an electron interacting with an atom is relatively small; therefore, the interactions of this primary agent of damage are sparse, and the ionizations produced are distant from each other. For this reason, x- and γ-rays are termed low-LET radiation.

In contrast to electromagnetic radiations, highly ionizing particulate radiations (e.g., α-particles and neutrons), having appreciable mass and/or charge, have a greater probability of interacting with matter. These types of radiations lose energy rapidly, producing many ionizations in a very short distance. Alpha particles and neutrons are high-LET radiations. Some average LET values for different types of radiation are given in Table 2–1 (refer to a text on radiation physics for a more complete discussion of LET).

Because of these differences in rates of energy loss, different LET radiations will produce different degrees of the same biologic response; equal doses of radiations of different LETs do not produce the same biologic response. A term relating the ability of radiations with different LETs to produce a specific biologic response is *relative biological effect (RBE)*. RBE is defined as the comparison of a dose of test radiation to the dose of 250 keV x-ray* that produces the same biologic response. This is expressed in the following formula:

$$RBE = \frac{\text{Dose in Gy from 250 keV x-ray}}{\substack{\text{Dose in Gy from another radiation} \\ \text{delivered under the same conditions} \\ \text{that produces the } same \text{ biologic effect.}}}$$

Note that the biologic response, *not* the dose of radiation, is the constant. What is actually measured is the biologic effectiveness of radiations of different LETs.

Although the relationship between LET and RBE has been discussed in simple terms, it is much more complex. RBE does provide useful information concerning the biologic effectiveness of different types of radiation, but it must be carefully used. RBE is a meaningful value if both the test system used and the biologic end point measured are identical. One of the major problems encountered in RBE determinations is that as radiation travels through matter, losing energy, the LET increases after each interaction until the ionizing particle finally stops; therefore, RBE also changes. For this reason, systems and end points must be carefully chosen.

RADIATION AND CELLULAR TARGETS

As stated previously, there are critical sites in the cell that, if damaged, have a higher probability of resulting in lethality than damage in other sites, regardless of the mechanism of damage (direct or indirect). In relationship to cell killing, this forms the basis for the term "targets."

As discussed in Chapter 1, the cell consists of many different molecules (e.g., enzymes, proteins, RNA, DNA) and organelles (e.g., mitochondria and ribosomes). All these molecules and organelles have specific functions to perform; however, they all have one common purpose—to work together and keep the cell alive. Each structure and molecule in the cell is important, but the number of these may vary. Many of the same enzymes may be present, but not all may play a role in the life of the cell at all times. Other molecules such as DNA are present only in the necessary amounts; thus, all are necessary for the

---

*250 keV x-ray is the *standard* for determining RBE because of its widespread use at the time the concept of RBE was adopted. Today, although cobalt 60 is more widely used, 250 keV x-ray remains the standard radiation for determining RBE.

proper functioning and life of the cell. These latter molecules can be considered critical molecules in the cell.

The existence of critical molecules and their importance in maintaining cellular integrity implies that damage to these molecules can be of far greater consequence to the cell than damage to molecules of which many are present. If more than the necessary number of molecules are present than are needed for normal functioning, and a few of these are damaged, one of the "extra" molecules can replace the damaged one and the cell will continue to function normally. However, if a critical molecule is damaged, this may present a life-threatening situation to the cell because there is no "extra" molecule present that can continue the function of the damaged one.

When ionizing radiation interacts with or within a short distance around one of these critical molecules, the name given to this sensitive area is "target." Target must not be interpreted as indicating selective interaction of radiation with a specific cellular site. This is certainly not the case, because all ionizing radiation interactions are random events with no specificity or selectivity for the site of interaction. The term target is based solely on the assumption that a random ionization occurring in this area will have greater consequences to the cell than an ionizing event occurring in another part of the cell.

Although this "target" has eluded positive identification, overwhelming data indicates that the nucleus is much more sensitive to radiation damage than the cytoplasm, thus implying that the target for radiation is a nuclear constituent. Since DNA is the molecule in the nucleus that controls all cellular activities, logically, an alteration in DNA can be assumed to present more serious consequences to the life of the cell than an alteration in other cellular constituents, such as enzymes or water molecules. Therefore, DNA is the most likely target for radiation action.

RADIATION EFFECTS ON DNA

As discussed above, overwhelming experimental data indicate that DNA is the most likely target in the cell for radiation. Before preceding with a discussion of the types of damage that have been observed, it is important to emphasize two points: (1) much of the damage in DNA can be, and is, *repaired* by the cell, and (2) all types of DNA damage are not equal in terms of their biologic significance.

With these two points in mind, then, radiation damage to DNA can be divided into four categories:

1. Base damage—change or loss of a base.
2. Single-strand breaks (SSB)—break in the backbone of one chain of the DNA molecule.
3. Double-strand break (DSB)—break in both chains of the DNA molecule.
4. Crosslinks—either within the DNA molecule (intrastrand) or from one molecule to another (DNA-interstrand or DNA-protein).

Base Damage

The loss or change of a base on the DNA chain results in an alteration of the base sequence. Since it is the sequence of these bases that stores and transmits genetic information, this can be of major consequence to the cell. Regardless of the severity of the consequences, loss or change of a base is considered a type of mutation.

Single-Strand Breaks

Breaks in just one of the strands of DNA molecules have been measured experimentally in cells in vitro and in vivo, but have been found to be relatively inconsequential in terms of cell killing. Thus, although single-strand breaks do occur as a result of irradiation, it is obvious that these are most likely efficiently repaired, with little, if any, long-term consequences to the cell.

Double-Strand Breaks

Breaks in both chains, or backbones, of the DNA, if they are in proximity, can have a significant impact on the cell. This type of damage is likely to be more difficult for the cell to repair accurately. (If the two breaks are not adjacent, they essentially are single-strand breaks.) Unlike single-strand breaks, double-strand breaks do show a reasonable correlation with cell killing. If repair does not take place, the DNA chains can separate, with greater consequence to the life of the cell.

Crosslinking

In addition to breakage of the DNA strands, radiation can produce covalent crosslinks involving DNA. An *intra*strand crosslink can be formed between two regions of the same DNA strand. Alternatively, *inter*strand crosslinks can be produced either between the two complementary DNA strands or between completely different DNA molecules. Finally, DNA molecules can become covalently linked to a protein molecule (DNA-protein crosslink). The importance of these lesions in cell killing is unclear, although they may be important if not repaired properly by the cell.

A schematic of some possible lesions in DNA is shown in Figure 2–2. It is not within the scope of the text to discuss in greater detail radiation-induced changes in DNA; however, it is important to realize the possible implications to the cell of damage to this structure. Radiation interaction with DNA does not always mean that permanent damage occurs in the cell; much of this damage can be, and probably is, repaired. Although the exact mechanism of this repair is unknown in mammalian cells, it is known that efficient repair of DNA damage occurs as long as the integrity of the undamaged chain is intact.

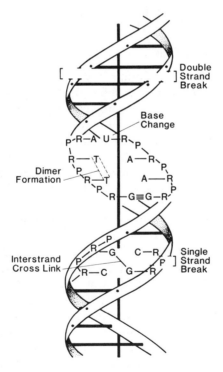

FIG 2–2.
Some possible lesions in DNA. (Courtesy of Dr Raymond E Meyn and Dr Ron Humphrey, M D Anderson Cancer Center.)

RADIATION EFFECTS ON CHROMOSOMES

Although changes in DNA can have serious implications for a cell, radiation-induced changes in a chromosome resulting in structural changes (breakage) of the chromosome are equally serious. Admittedly, changes in the DNA molecule are reflected in the chromosome; however, DNA changes are discrete and do not necessarily result in visible structural chromosome changes.

Some chromosome breaks produced by radiation can be observed microscopically during the subsequent postirradiation cell division and are evident during metaphase and anaphase, when the chromosomes are shortened and visible. The events that have occurred prior to this time can only be inferred, since they are not visible. What are observable are the consequences of these events, the gross or visible changes in chromosome structure. Radiation-induced chromosome breaks can occur in both somatic cells and in germ cells, and can be transmitted during mitosis and meiosis, respectively.

General Chromosome Effects

The overall result of radiation interacting with a chromosome is breakage of the chromosome, thereby producing two or more chromosomal fragments, each having a broken end. These broken ends have the important capability of being able to join with other broken ends, usually with the first broken end encountered, possibly forming new chromosomes. These new chromosomes may or may not appear structurally different from the chromosome prior to irradiation.

The gross structural changes in a chromosome after irradiation are interchangeably termed *aberrations, lesions,* or *anomalies.* A distinction is made between a *chromosome aberration* and a *chromatid aberration.* During the S-phase of the cell cycle, the chromosome lays down an exact duplicate of itself. These two like chromosomes are termed *sister chromatids.* Chromatid aberrations are those produced in individual chromatids when irradiation occurs *after* DNA synthesis. Because only one chromatid of a pair has been damaged, only one daughter cell will be affected. Chromosome aberrations, on the other hand, are produced when irradiation occurs before DNA synthesis. A resultant break will be replicated if repair is not completed before the initiation of DNA synthesis. In this case, both chromatids will exhibit the break, and both daughter cells will inherit a damaged chromatid.

Because of its randomness, radiation may produce a variety of structural changes, some of which are:

1. A single break in one chromosome or chromatid.
2. A single break in separate chromosomes or chromatids.
3. Two or more breaks in the same chromosome or chromatid.
4. "Stickiness," or clumping, of the chromosomes.

The general consequence to the cell of these structural changes may be one of the following:

1. The broken ends may rejoin with no visible damage. This process, termed *restitution*, results in no damage to the cell because the chromosome has been restored to its pre-irradiated condition. Ninety-five percent of single chromosome breaks are believed to heal by restitution.
2. Loss of part of the chromosome or chromatid at the next mitosis, giving rise to an aberration. This process is termed *deletion*. The resultant aberration is an acentric fragment.
3. Rearrangement of the broken ends, which can produce a grossly distorted chromosome. Some examples are ring chromosomes, dicentric chromosomes, and anaphase bridges.
4. Rearrangement of the broken ends without visible chromosomal damage; the genetic material has been rearranged, but the chromosome looks fine. Examples are translocations and inversions. Such changes, although perhaps not immediately lethal to the cell, result in rearrangement of the genes on the chromosomes, thereby changing the inheritable characteristics of the cell. In this case, a mutation has been produced.

Structural Changes

Acentric Fragments and Dicentric Rings.—A break in the arms of two different chromosomes before replication (or in the arm of one chromosome which then replicates) results in four chromosome fragments, two with centromeres and two without centromeres, each having broken sticky ends. If restitution does not occur, the two chromatids without a centromere may join, forming an *acentric* chromatid, and the two chromatids with centromeres may join to form a *dicentric* chromatid (Fig 2–3).

The consequences of this type of damage are visible during mitosis (Fig 2–4). The acentric chromatid will not attach to the mitotic spindle because of the absence of a centromere. Therefore, the amount of genetic information carried on the acentric chromatid will not be transmitted to the daughter cell.

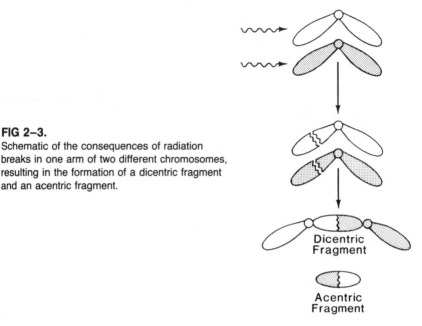

FIG 2–3.
Schematic of the consequences of radiation breaks in one arm of two different chromosomes, resulting in the formation of a dicentric fragment and an acentric fragment.

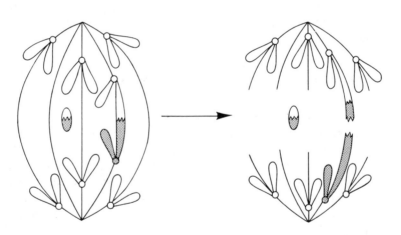

FIG 2–4.
Fates of the dicentric and acentric fragments in Fig 2–3. The dicentric fragment attaches to the mitotic spindle but migrates to opposite poles of the cell *(left)*, ultimately breaking again *(right)*. The acentric fragment does not attach to the spindle, resulting in loss of genetic information.

The dicentric chromatid will attach to the spindle; however, the two centromeres will orient the chromatid toward opposite poles of the cell. During anaphase, one centromere will pull the chromatid toward one pole and the other centromere will pull it toward the other pole. As the centromeres continue to migrate to opposite poles of the cell, the chromatid section between them (the junction site of the original broken ends) will be stretched. Eventually, the chromatid will break again, although not necessarily at the point of fusion of the original broken ends. Each chromosome will be drawn into one of the daughter nuclei and the same process can be repeated, since a chromosome with a broken end is still present. If this process continues through many divisions, a major part or even the entire chromosome may eventually be lost from the cell.

The ultimate result of a single chromosome break, then, is loss of genetic information from both daughter cells, either in the form of a whole chromosome or part of a chromosome, and transmission of incomplete genetic information to both daughter cells.

Whereas a single break in a chromosome before replication will affect both daughter cells, a single break in a chromatid after DNA replication will affect only one daughter cell. The ultimate result in this situation will be the same—loss of genetic information—but the damage will be transmitted to only one daughter cell.

Ring Chromosomes.—Due to the random nature of radiation, an ionizing event can occur in each arm of the same chromosome. Again, three fragments are formed: two with only one broken end and one with two broken ends. In this case, the fragment with two broken ends will contain the centromere, and the fragments with one broken end each will be acentric.

A break in each arm of a chromosome can result in very bizarre and unusual chromosome aberrations, an example of which is a ring chromosome. The two broken ends of the fragment with the centromere may move about, coming in close contact. If this occurs, these broken ends follow the rule of all broken ends—they join, forming a ring (Fig 2–5). When DNA synthesis occurs, the ring will be replicated and will be transmitted to each daughter cell during anaphase, because each chromosome has a centromere.

As the broken ends of the fragment with the centromere are moving about in the cell, they may twist before joining, forming a twisted ring. When DNA synthesis occurs, again, the ring is synthesized; however, in this case the replicated rings are intertwined so that separation at the next anaphase is impossible. One daughter cell will be deficient in

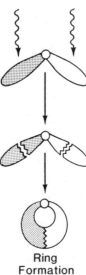

FIG 2–5.
One possible consequence of breaks in both arms of a chromosome by radiation is that the broken arms join to form a ring, while the remaining fragments join but are left without a centromere (acentric fragment).

Ring
Formation

Acentric
Fragment

one entire chromosome, and the other daughter cell will have one too many chromosomes. In this situation both daughter cells will be seriously affected.

One other consequence of a break in each arm of the same chromosome is the formation of an acentric fragment, which, with its attendant genetic information, will be deleted from the cell, as described previously.

Many other chromosome aberrations have been observed after irradiation, including such bizarre configurations as star and propellor chromosomes, but the mechanism of these formations is outside the scope of this text. However, it is likely that all of these represent lethal aberrations that result in cell death. Suffice it to say that the more chromosomes in a cell that sustain double breaks, the greater the number and the more complex will be the resultant aberrations exhibited by the cell. All of the described changes and many others have been observed in the cells of patients undergoing radiation therapy, as well as in individuals occupationally exposed to radiation (Fig 2–6).

Chromosome Stickiness.—Another phenomenon observed in chromosomes after irradiation, stickiness, occurs in cells already in division at the time of radiation. At metaphase, and particularly during anaphase, the chromosomes appear to be clumped together. Although the mechanism causing this type of damage is still unknown, one possibility is alteration of the chemical composition of the protein component of the chromosome by radiation, allowing the chromosomes to adhere to each other. The chromosomes cannot separate at metaphase and anaphase and form bridges between the two opposite poles of the cell. This results in errors in the transmission of genetic information to the daughter cells.

Changes in the Sequence of Genetic Information: Translocations and Inversions

Although the gross structural changes described above can have an immediate and drastic impact on the cell, other more discrete chromosome changes can occur, which, although not immediately lethal, are equally damaging to the cell. Two of these are translocations and inversions. Both of these processes require two breaks, either in the same or different chromosomes. The overall outcome of these two pro-

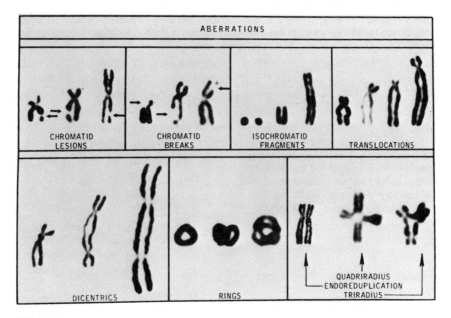

FIG 2–6.
Photomicrograph of chromosomes from patients undergoing radiation therapy illustrating many and varied aberrations. (From of Berdjis CC: *Pathology of Irradiation.* Baltimore, Williams & Wilkins, 1971. Used by permission.)

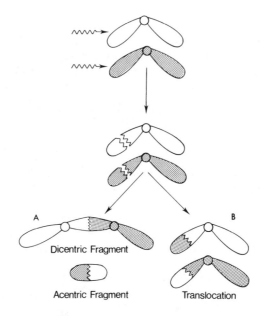

FIG 2–7.

Two different chromosomes *(top)* may each sustain a single break in one arm *(center)*, resulting in **A,** formation of dicentric and acentric fragments, or **B,** translocation of genetic information between the two. In the latter process, two complete chromosomes are formed. Note, however, the exchange of chromosome parts.

FIG 2–8.

Two breaks occurring in the same arm of a chromosome *(top* and *middle)* may result in **A,** deletion of the fragment between the two breaks, or **B,** inversion of this fragment, illustrated by the change in the positions of the break lines.

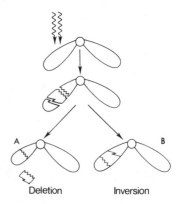

cesses is to change the sequence of the genes on the chromosome (Figs 2–7 and 2–8).

The consequences of these changes will be dependent on the cell type in which they occur. In a somatic cell, a change of gene sequence will not necessarily result in major (life-threatening) consequences to the cell because the necessary number of chromosomes is present. This does not, however, exclude the possibility that the functions these genes control may be altered because of their rearrangement on the chromosome.

The consequences to the cell of these rearrangements will be dependent on the number of genes and bases in the inverted section and the functions they controlled. The linear sequence of bases on DNA is the ultimate control of all cellular functions; therefore, it is not unrealistic to presume that a change in sequence can be of major consequence to the cell.

An example might help to clarify the potential damage to a cell of this type of chromosome damage. Protein synthesis is "ordered" by the linear sequence of bases on DNA, the sequence of bases forming a "code." An inversion or translocation changes the order, and therefore the code, carried by the DNA, resulting in the production of proteins that are different from the proteins originally coded for. These new proteins may or may not be usable by the cell. More importantly, this change may order "nonsense" proteins the cell cannot utilize, resulting in decreased amounts of precursor molecules available as building blocks for many substances necessary for life.

Another important point to remember is that different genes on the same chromosome are not necessarily independent of each other. A gene at one end of a chromosome may control the activities of a gene at the other end, which in turn controls the function of a gene elsewhere on the same chromosome. Inversions and translocations can upset this interrelationship between genes at different sites on the chromosome and render all of them either nonfunctional or always functional.

Translocations and inversions in a germ cell can be of major consequence, particularly if occurring in a gamete that plays a part in conception. The altered chromosome can be transmitted to succeeding generations and, depending on the severity of the damage, may result in either nonviable offspring or offspring that, although surviving into adulthood, may have gross malformations or impaired functions. Of course, the possibility also exists that the effects of the damaged chromosome will never be exhibited in the offspring.

Implications to Humans

Although the implications to humans of DNA and chromosome damage will be discussed thoroughly in a later chapter, it may be of value to put these into perspective at this point. A change in a chromosome means corresponding changes in DNA. Changes in DNA, either an alteration in the amount of DNA resulting from a deletion, or an alteration in the sequence of bases on the DNA molecule, result in a change in genetic information in the cell. These changes in genetic information are termed mutations.

It is not always feasible to determine the consequences of mutations to the cell. Some of the consequences will be major, such as death of the cell. Others, however are not detectable and do not result in death of the cell. In fact, these discrete changes, difficult, if not impossible, to detect, can be of great importance to humans and to the general population.

The type of cell (somatic or germ cell) in which the change occurs has important implications. Though mutations in somatic cells have consequences for that individual, they do not have an effect on the general population. Germ cell mutations, on the other hand, do affect the general population because the cell carrying the mutation can play a role in conception and affect future generations.

RADIATION EFFECTS ON OTHER CELLULAR CONSTITUENTS

Because of their obvious importance to the life of the cell, much attention has been, and continues to be, focused on DNA and chromosomes. However, other molecules and organelles in the cell also exhibit radiation effects. Radiation has been observed to cause chain breakage in carbohydrates, structural changes in proteins, and alterations in the activity of enzymes. Lipids also exhibit changes after irradiation. Although damage to these molecules does not appear to be as important as damage to DNA, more knowledge is necessary concerning not only the effects of radiation on these molecules, but also the implications of this damage to the cell.

Chromosomes are not the only organelles affected by radiation. Permeability of the cell membrane is altered after irradiation, affecting the transport function of the membrane and its ability to keep molecules in or out of the cell. Alteration of membranes by radiation can also affect organelles in the cell that are membrane-bound, e.g., mitochondria and lysosomes. The effect of radiation on cell organelles and the role of damage to these structures in terms of the cellular response to radiation is a subject that requires further study.

REFERENCES

1. Alexander P, Charles BA: Energy transfer in macromolecules exposed to ionizing radiation. *Nature (London)* 1954; 173:578.
2. Alper T, Cramp WA, Hornsey S, et al (eds): Cellular Repair of Radiation Damage: Mechanisms and Modifying Agents, Proceedings of the 11th LH Gray Conference. *Br J Cancer* 1984; 49 (suppl VI).
3. Amarose AP, et al: Residual chromosome aberrations in female cancer patients after irradiation therapy. *Exp Molec Pathol* 1967; 7:58.
4. Bacq AM, Alexander P: *Fundamentals of Radiobiology*, ed 2. New York, Pergamon Press, 1961.
5. Bender M: Induced aberrations in human chromosomes. *Am J Pathol* 1963; 43:26a.
6. Berdjis CC: *Pathology of Irradiation*. Baltimore, Williams & Wilkins, 1971.
7. Blois MS Jr: *Free Radicals in Biological Systems*. New York, Academic Press, 1961.
8. Bonura J, Smith KC: The involvement of indirect effects in cell-killing and DNA double strand breakage in γ-irradiated *Escherichia coli* K-12. *Int J Radiat Biol* 1976; 29:293–296.
9. Carlson JG: An analysis of x-ray induced single breaks in neuroblast chromosomes of the grasshopper (*Chortophaga viridifasciata*). *Proc Natl Acad Sci* 1941; 27:42.
10. Chu EHY, et al: Types and frequencies of human chromosome aberrations induced by x-rays. *Proc Natl Acad Sci* 1961; 47:830.
11. Collins A, Downes CS, Johnson RT (eds): *DNA Repair and Its Inhibition*. Oxford, IRL Press, Nucleic Acid Symposium Series No 13, 1984.
12. Dewey WC, Humphrey RM: Restitution of radiation induced chromosomal damage in Chinese hamster cells related to the cell's life cycle. *Exp Cell Res* 1964; 35:262.
13. Ebert M, Howard A: *Radiation Effects in Physics, Chemistry, and Biology*. Amsterdam: North Holland Publishing Co, 1963.
14. Errera M, Forssberg A: *Mechanisms in Radiobiology*. New York, Academic Press, 1960.
15. Evans HJ: Chromosome aberrations induced by ionizing radiation. *Int Rev Cytol* 1962; 13:221.
16. Giles NH, Tobias CA: Effect of linear energy transfer on radiation induced chromosome aberrations in *Tradescantia* microspores. *Science* 1954; 120:993.
17. Hall EJ: *Radiobiology for the Radiologist*, ed 3. Philadelphia, JB Lippincott, 1988.
18. Kaufman BP: Chromosome aberrations induced in animal cells by ionizing radiations, in Hollander A (ed): *Radiation Biology*, vol 6. New York, McGraw-Hill Book Co, 1954, p 627.
19. Lea DE: *Actions of Radiation on Living Cells*, ed 2. Cambridge, Cambridge University Press, 1956.

20. Little JB: Cellular effects of ionizing radiation. *N Engl J Med* 1968; 278:308.
21. MacCardle RC, Congdon TC: Mitochondrial changes in hepatic cells in x-irradiated mice. *Am J Pathol* 1955; 31:725.
22. Moore R: Ionizing radiations in chromosomes. *J Coll Radiol Australia* 1965; 9:272.
23. Müller HJ: On the relation between chromosome changes and gene mutations. *Brookhaven Symposium on Biology* 1956; 8:126.
24. Sax K: An analysis of x-ray induced chromosomal aberrations in *Tradescantia*. *Genetics* 1940; 25:41.
25. Sax K: Chromosome aberrations induced by x-rays. *Genetics* 1938; 23:494.
26. Sax K: The effect of ionizing radiation on chromosomes. *Q Rev Biol* 1957; 32:15.
27. Simic MG, Grossman L, Upton AC (eds): *Mechanisms of DNA Damage and Repair.* New York, Plenum Press, 1986.
28. Srb V: Immediate and short time changes in cell permeability after x-irradiation. *Radiat Res* 1964; 21:308.
29. Ward JF: Biochemistry of DNA lesions. *Radiat Res* 1985; 104:S103–S111.
30. Wolff S: Chromosome aberrations in the cell cycle. *Radiat Res* 1968; 33:609.
31. Wolff S: *Radiation-Induced Chromosome Aberrations.* New York, Columbia University Press, 1963.
32. Wolff S, Luippold ME: Metabolism and chromosome break rejoining. *Science* 1955; 122:231.
33. Zirkle RE: Partial cell irradiation. *Adv Biol Med Phys* 1957; 5:103.

Chapter 3 —————————————

Cellular Response to Radiation

—————————————

As early as 11 years after the discovery of radiation, radiation injuries were reported in occupationally exposed persons. Fascinated with these "magic" rays which allowed them to see inside the living body and unaware of the dangers involved, many people used radiation indiscriminately. One of the first reported cases of radiation damage involved a physician who had lost his hair because he had allowed another physician to repeatedly use x-rays to "see" inside his skull! Reports of radiation injuries led to observation and investigation of the biologic effects of radiation. By studying responses such as skin erythema and hair loss, scientists proposed basic postulates concerning the responses of different cell populations to radiation. It was not until the 1920s, however, that techniques were developed to study individual cells and their response to radiation. The ingenuity and imagination of these early investigators in developing these techniques is striking; many techniques used today are based on these early investigations.

There are many ways to study the responses of cells to radiation, both in vivo (in the living organism) and in vitro (in glassware). Tissue culture (growing of animal and human cells in a bottle or tube by providing nutrients) is an extremely useful in vitro tool for studying the response of single cell types to radiation because vasculature and other physiologic factors present in the living organism do not contribute to the response.

Studies may be performed on asynchronous populations of cells; that is, the population being studied contains cells in all four phases of the cell cycle (G_1, S, G_2, and M). Other studies are performed on synchronous populations, necessitating techniques that place all cells in a given phase of the cell cycle at a given time. Dividing populations of cells in the body are asynchronous; therefore, the first method more nearly simulates the in vivo situation. The second method permits observation of the response of cells in each phase of the cell cycle.

One of the classic studies in radiation biology involved the construction of the first survival curve for mammalian cells by Puck and Marcus. These investigators grew HeLa cells (derived from human carcinoma of the cervix) in tissue culture and kept them alive for many generations. In fact, the first culture was started in 1956, and today it is possible to purchase HeLa cells from biologic supply companies. Puck and Marcus exposed the cells to various doses of radiation and observed the ability of the cells to reproduce. Other investigators (Withers; McCulloch and Till) have developed techniques to construct cell survival curves using in vivo systems, such as the skin and hemopoietic systems.

Because the response of the individual cell cannot be observed in all systems in vivo, this chapter will deal with responses that have been observed in vitro and in appropriate in vivo systems.

FATE OF IRRADIATED CELLS

One of three things can happen to a cell after irradiation:

1. It can be delayed from going through division; appropriately, the term used to define this response is *division delay*.
2. It can die before it divides, during interphase. This response is also appropriately named *interphase death*.
3. It can die when attempting mitosis; this response is termed *reproductive failure*.

Division delay occurs in both nonlethally and lethally damaged cells. Interphase death and reproductive failure, which, by definition, occur only in lethally damaged cells, represent two fundamentally different modes of cell death.

Division Delay

This cellular response to radiation involves mitosis. In dividing asynchronous populations of cells, a certain proportion of cells will be in mitosis at any one time. The ratio of the number of cells in mitosis at any one time to the total number of cells in the population is termed the *mitotic index*. If this ratio is plotted on graph paper, with mitotic index plotted on the y axis and time plotted on the x axis, the mitotic index remains relatively constant—as some cells are completing mitosis, others are entering prophase, maintaining the mitotic index at a status quo.

Irradiation of the population disturbs this ratio of mitotic to nonmitotic cells (Fig 3–1). Cells in mitosis at the time of irradiation complete division, but those about to enter division are delayed in G_2. The mitotic index, therefore, decreases for a period of time as some cells are stopped from proceeding through mitosis at their appointed time. If the dose is low enough, these cells recover from this delay and proceed through mitosis—resulting in an increased number of cells in mitosis, appropriately termed *mitotic overshoot*. During this time, cells entering mitosis consist of two classes: those normally progressing through mitosis that were not delayed by irradiation and those that were delayed by irradiation. This cellular response to radiation is termed *division* or *mitotic delay*.

Canti and Spear observed division delay in chick fibroblasts in tissue culture irradiated with varying doses of γ-rays from a radium source (Fig 3–2). Low doses (0.5 Gy) produced a negligible effect on mitotic index; as dose increased (0.83 and 3 Gy), the response became more pronounced, i.e., both the length and magnitude of the delay were increased. The mitotic overshoot increased in magnitude with these effects, the length and magnitude of the overshoot reflecting the delay.

The overshoot was followed by a return of the mitotic index to its pre-irradiated (100%) value after exposure to low doses (0.5 and 0.83 Gy). However, after higher doses, the mitotic index fell below the pre-irradiated value and remained there. At these doses a third mechanism of damage was operational: the cells divided but died after division. This response, termed *reproductive failure*, will be discussed in a later section.

A more dramatic response was observed following a dose of 10 Gy.

PREIRRADIATION   POSTIRRADIATION

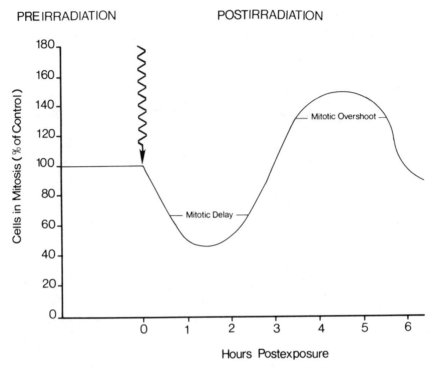

FIG 3–1.
Effects of radiation on an asynchronous, dividing population of cells. Prior to irradiation, the
mitotic index remains at a constant value; radiation *(wavy arrow)* disturbs this constant ratio
of cells, effecting a decrease in the number of cells in mitosis *(mitotic delay)*, which may be
overcome (depending on dose) to produce an increase in the number of cells in mitosis at
any time *(mitotic overshoot)*.

Not only were the length and magnitude of delay greatly increased, but
no mitotic overshoot occurred, indicating the cells apparently were not
able to overcome the block imposed by the radiation, and therefore died
before division *(interphase death)*.

Division delay can be induced in cells by doses as low as 0.1 Gy;
0.5 Gy to human kidney cells in tissue culture results in division delay.
An opportunity to observe division delay in vivo occurred when five
people were overexposed to radiation in a reactor accident (Y-12 accident). Dose estimates to these individuals ranged from 0.5 to 2 Gy.
Observation of cells in the bone marrow of these individuals showed
a progressive decrease in mitotic index, approaching zero on the 4th
day postirradiation.

The underlying cause of mitotic delay is unknown. Some theories
proposed to explain this phenomenon are (1) a chemical involved in

division is altered by irradiation; (2) proteins necessary for mitosis are not synthesized; and (3) DNA synthesis does not progress at the same rate following irradiation.

In summary, division delay is a dose-dependent phenomenon; the decrease in mitotic index and the length of the delay are a function of dose. At low doses, the duration of delay and decrease in mitotic index are much less than at higher doses. The mitotic overshoot reflects the ability of the cells to overcome the radiation-induced block and proceed through mitosis along with unaffected cells, indicating that the process is reversible. Division delay occurs only at specific points in the cell cycle, in G_2 and at the beginning of DNA synthesis. Essentially, radiation acts as a synchronizing agent by selectively affecting cells in these two stages of the cell cycle, delaying their progression through mitosis. This response will be discussed in the next chapter.

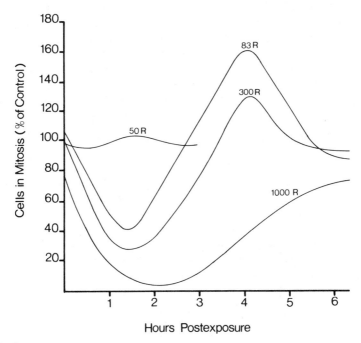

FIG 3–2.
Experimental findings by Canti and Spear illustrating the dose dependence of mitotic delay. Doses in R are equivalent to 0.5 Gy, 0.83 Gy, 3 Gy and 10 Gy. (From Canti RG, Spear FG: The effect of gamma irradiation on cell division in tissue culture in vitro, Part II. *Proc R Soc Lond [Biol]* 1929; 105:93. Used by permission.)

Interphase Death

A second response of the cell to radiation is death before it enters mitosis. This response is called *interphase death*; synonymous terms are *nonmitotic* or *nondivision death*. Interphase death can occur in cells that do not divide and are long-lived (e.g., adult nerve), and in rapidly dividing cells (e.g., blood cell precursors in the bone marrow), and has been observed after irradiation of oocytes, erythroblasts, and cancer cells. Recent studies have shown that interphase death occurs in nondividing cells in tissues that are of importance in radiotherapy. The prototypical cell that has long been known to die after low doses of irradiation via this mechanism is the small mature lymphocyte, a nondividing cell. More recently, interphase death has been identified as the mechanism whereby cells die in the serous acini of parotid glands (salivary glands) and lachrymal glands (the glands of the eye that produce tears).

The radiation dose for interphase death is dependent on the cell: lymphocytes exhibit interphase death at doses less than 0.50 Gy, mouse spermatogonia at 0.25 Gy, and parotid cells after a single dose of about 9.0 Gy. Although the relationship between interphase death, cell type, and dose is poorly understood, in general, rapidly dividing, undifferentiated (radiosensitive) cells exhibit interphase death at lower doses than nondividing, differentiated (radioresistant) cells. The one exception to this generalization is the lymphocyte, (usually a nondividing cell), which undergoes interphase death at very low doses.

Morphologically, interphase death is not a degenerative process like cellular necrosis in which the whole cell disintegrates, although these two modes of cell destruction share some common nuclear changes, such as fragmentation. In interphase death the cell condenses and breaks up into pieces, but the cytoplasmic organelles remain intact. These pieces are then phagocytosed by other cells.

Interphase death is not a unique effect of irradiation on cells, but is a general phenomenon that occurs spontaneously in healthy as well as diseased tissues. Termed *apoptosis*, which comes from Greek and means "falling off," as leaves from a tree, this process appears to be programmed self-destruction. A familiar example of apoptosis is the loss of the tail by a tadpole during metamorphosis.

The mechanism of interphase death and apoptosis is obscure. It is unrelated to mitosis, as it is not an unsuccessful attempt by the cell to divide. Recently, it has been suggested that this mode of cell death may be due to changes in the plasma membrane, with accompanying imbalances in extracellular and intracellular salts, e.g., Na, K, and Ca.

Reproductive Failure

A third type of cellular response to radiation is a decrease in the percentage of cells surviving after irradiation that have retained their reproductive integrity, i.e., are capable of reproducing. This is termed *reproductive failure* and is defined as the inability of the cell to undergo repeated divisions after irradiation. By this definition, all cells that cannot *repeatedly* divide and produce a large number of progeny are considered nonsurvivors or "dead," even though they may still be technically alive (metabolizing or capable of a limited number of divisions). This concept can be understood in terms of the target theory (Chapter 2). The ability of a cell to reproduce is directly related to the integrity of the chromosomes. If it is assumed that chromosomes (or DNA) are the critical sites (targets) in the cell and that only an ionizing event occurring in the target is responsible for cell death, then damage to the chromosomes may result in death of the cell. However, much of this damage can be, and usually ís, repaired. If it is not repaired, the cell may still retain some ability to divide, doing so one or more times following irradiation. These cellular responses to radiation are summarized in Table 3–1.

Puck and Marcus experimentally quantitated reproductive failure by exposing human cells (HeLa) to various doses of radiation and counting the number of colonies formed by these irradiated cells. They graphically expressed the ability of cells to reproduce after different doses of radiation in the form of a semilogarithmic curve, where dose is plotted on a linear scale (x axis) and surviving fraction on a logarithmic scale (y axis). This curve, illustrated in Figure 3–3 is termed a *cell survival curve*.

SURVIVAL CURVES FOR MAMMALIAN CELLS

A cell survival curve describes the relationship between radiation dose and proportion of cells that survive. Critical to an understanding of this relationship between dose and cell kill is the appreciation of the randomness of the deposition of energy by radiation. Some cells will sustain more than one "hit," some will be hit only once, and some will not be hit at all. Thus, if each cell in a population requires one hit to be killed, for a given increment in dose, the *proportion* of cells killed will remain the same but the absolute number of cells killed will vary, as shown in Table 3–2. This table illustrates the exponential function of the response of cells exposed to equal dose increments. Note the same dose (5.0 Gy) always kills the same proportion (50%) of cells, but

TABLE 3–1.
Types of Cell Damage

Type	Changes	Dose	Mechanism
Interphase death	Normal nuclear architecture disappears	High in most cases, except for lymphocytes	May be biochemical
Division delay	Lowered mitotic index; delayed mitosis	Exhibited by dividing cells; dose-dependent, degree of response varies with dose	Unknown: change in a chemical involved in division; proteins are not synthesized; DNA synthesis is affected
Reproductive failure	Loss of reproductive integrity; cells cannot undergo repeated division	Exhibited by dividing cells; dose-dependent, high doses affect greater number	Damage to genomic DNA

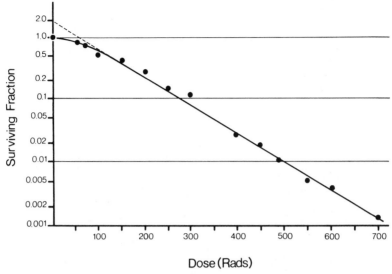

Dose (Rads)

FIG 3–3.
Illustration of the survival curve determined by Puck and Marcus. Below 150 rad (1.5 Gy) the curve exhibits a shoulder region, becoming exponential at higher doses. (From Puck TT, Marcus TI: Action of x-rays on mammalian cells. *J Exp Med* 1956; 103:653. Used by permission.)

the absolute number of cells killed varies. This type of data indicates a logarithmic relationship between dose and surviving fraction. These data would form a straight line on a semi-logarithmic plot (Fig 3–4) and indicate that cell kill is an exponential function of dose. Two doses of 5.0 Gy actually inactivate only 75%, not 100%, of the original population. If two doses of 5.0 Gy did inactivate 100% of the population, the response would be linear, not exponential.*

Few mammalian cells irradiated with sparsely ionizing x- or γ-rays exhibit this survival curve shape. Rather, the survival curve for mam-

TABLE 3–2.
Typical Data Relating Dose and Surviving Fraction*

Original Cell Number	Dose Delivered (Gy)	Fraction (%) Cells Killed	Number of Cells Killed
100,000	5	50	50,000
50,000	5	50	25,000
25,000	5	50	12,500
12,500	5	50	6,250
6,250	5	50	3,125

*This is the same principle that describes the decay of a radioactive isotope.

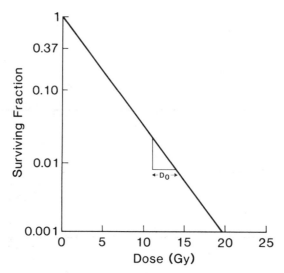

FIG 3–4.
Survival curve for bacteria *(Escherichia coli)*, showing that in this system survival is a simple exponential function of dose.

malian cells exposed to different doses of x- or γ-rays exhibits a broad initial shoulder, followed by a steep, straight portion (the survival curve in Figure 3–3 is typical for mammalian cells). In the shoulder region, equal increases in dose do not cause a corresponding equal decrease in surviving fraction. In other words, in the example in Figure 3–3, doses less than 2 Gy are inefficient in producing cell death. This region of the cell survival curve implies that, in mammalian cells, damage must be accumulated before the cell dies. If damage did not have to be accumulated, each dose of radiation, starting with the lowest, would be as efficient as the next in causing cell death. This curve then would be a straight line from its origin on the y axis at 0 dose and 100% surviving fraction (see Fig 3–4). After higher doses (>2 Gy in Fig 3–3), the curve does form a straight line on a logarithmic plot; cell kill is now an exponential function of dose.

In recent years the shoulder region of the survival curve has been examined more closely and it is now known that survival also is exponential over the initial "low-dose" region of the shoulder, after which it bends to form the shoulder. Both the initial and final ("high dose") regions of the survival curve are exponential; however, the two exponential regions of the survival curve have different slopes, i.e., the initial slope is generally more shallow than the final.

Two different mechanisms of cell killing have been suggested to describe the shape of this curve:

1. Lethal single-hit killing.
2. Interaction of a sufficient number of sublethal lesions to cause death.

The model most often used to describe the effects of these two types of lesions on cell killing is the target theory. The target theory states that there are n targets in a cell, all of which must be "hit" to kill the cell. If one target is not hit, the cell will survive and repair the damage. As the dose increases, however, more and more sublethal damage is accumulated and the cell dies. The final exponential shape of the survival curve is obtained when all cells have sustained $n - 1$ hits and the population now has only one target in each cell that must be hit to be killed. The initial slope in the shoulder region is more difficult to explain. After such low doses, it is unlikely that sufficient sublethal damage will be accumulated to kill the cell. Thus, cell killing must be by single-hit events.

DESCRIPTIONS OF "SHOULDERED" SURVIVAL CURVES

The cell survival curve can be defined by three graphic parameters: n (extrapolation number) and D_q (quasi-threshold dose), both of which refer to the shoulder region, and D_o dose, which refers to the terminal slope. A fourth term $1D_o$ is used to describe the initial exponential slope.

The extrapolation number n is determined by extrapolating the linear portion of the curve back to its intersection with the y axis (Fig 3–5). This term was originally referred to as the target number and was assumed to represent the number of targets that must be hit in each cell to cause cell death. However, objections arose over the use of the term "target," and it is now referred to as the extrapolation number. The n for mammalian cells ranges from two to ten.

The D_q defines the width of the shoulder region of the curve, and is the dose at which the extrapolation of the terminal portion of the curve intercepts the dose axis at 100% survival (i.e., surviving fraction of 1.0) (Fig 3–5). The point cannot be made too emphatically that D_q and n provide information only on the size of the shoulder and not its shape.

D_o is determined from the final exponential portion of the curve and is the reciprocal of the slope (1/slope) (Fig 3–5). This expression was derived mathematically from the target theory, and is defined as the dose that inactivates all but 37% of the population. D_o is an expression of radiosensitivity of a population. Cells with high D_o doses exhibit a shallow survival curve and are less sensitive (more resistant) than populations with low D_o doses, which give steep survival curves. D_o doses for different populations of mammalian cells vary between 1 and 2 Gy.

The three parameters are related by the expression

$$\text{Log}_e\ n = D_q/D_o$$

or

$$\text{Surviving Fraction (SF)} = ne^{-D/D_o}$$

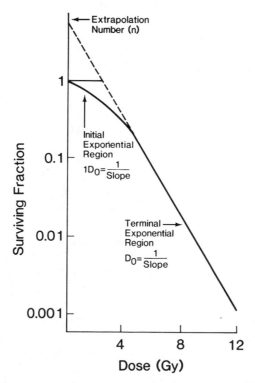

FIG 3–5.
A typical survival curve for mammalian cells exhibiting an initial shoulder followed by a terminal exponential region. The curve is characterized by an initial shoulder with some slope to it ($1D_o$), the terminal exponential slope (D_o), n (extrapolation number) and D_q (quasi-threshold dose). (Redrawn from Fletcher GH (ed): *Textbook of Radiotherapy,* ed 3. Philadelphia, Lea & Febiger, 1980, p 108.)

A second model, the linear quadratic model, has also been proposed to describe the survival curve for mammalian cells, but with only two parameters, α and β. This model assumes that there are two components to cell killing: (1) α, which is proportional to dose (D), and (2) β, which is proportional to dose squared (D^2). Survival is then expressed as

$$SF = \alpha D + \beta D^2$$

One interpretation of the parameters of this model is that α refers to single-hit killing and β to the interaction of lesions. Regardless of its mechanistic interpretation, the linear quadratic model provides a good empirical description of mammalian cell survival curves, particularly in the low-dose region.

The ratio of these two parameters, α/β, which has as units dose, has been shown to divide normal tissues into two categories based on their responses to dose fractionation. This has obvious importance to clinical radiotherapy and will be discussed further in Chapter 10.

Survival curves can be obtained from in vitro cultures of cell lines, as well as for certain tissues in vivo—those that contain proliferating cells that form a clone after irradiation. Survival curves can now be obtained for many normal tissues in vivo, e.g., crypt cells of the intestine, stem cells in the bone marrow, and epithelial cells in the skin.

In summary, three things happen in a population of cells after irradiation:

1. Some cells will receive no damage to a critical site and will be unaffected.
2. Some cells will accumulate enough damage to be lethal and will die in the next division.
3. Some cells will accumulate a degree of damage that is not lethal (sublethal) and which, given enough time, can be repaired, thus forming the shoulder. If more damage is received before the first damage is repaired, the two may interact to become lethal.

SURVIVAL CURVES AND REPAIR

It is well known that after sparsely ionizing radiations (e.g., x + γ) damage is repaired. This phenomenon has been demonstrated in many systems, including cells in culture, and in normal tissues and malignant tumors in experimental animals. Two types of repair have been defined, based on the type of experiment performed. The first, sublethal damage (SLD) repair, occurs when two doses are separated by time. Sublethal damage normally can be repaired unless another dose of radiation is added, in which case the effect becomes cumulative, resulting in cell death. The second, potentially lethal damage (PLD) repair, occurs when the postirradiation conditions are modified.

It is important to recognize that these are both operational definitions because little is known about either type of damage, where it actually occurs in the cell, and if the two are in any way related. However, they are important concepts to understanding cellular responses to radiation, and further explanation is warranted.

Sublethal Damage (SLD)

Sublethal damage and its repair were first described in cells grown in culture by Elkind and Sutton-Gilbert in 1960. Their investigations showed that when a given dose of radiation was divided into two equal doses (split dose) separated by various intervals of time, the surviving fraction of cells was larger than if the same total dose were given as a single dose (Fig 3–6). In addition, survival increased with time between the two doses, up to 2 hours, when survival reached a plateau that was four times higher than survival after this same total dose had been given as a single dose. No further increase in survival was observed after 2 hours in this cell line. The investigators suggested that the increase in repair was due to repair of sublethal damage.

Sublethal damage and its repair are measured experimentally in split-dose experiments and can be understood by a study of what happens to the survival curves in these experiments. An example of the survival curves from a split-dose experiment is shown in Figure 3–7. The first dose reduces survival to the terminal exponential portion of the curve. If sufficient time elapses between the two doses, the surviving cells respond as if they were never irradiated, i.e., the survival curve for the surviving cells is exactly the same shape and the shoulder has been repeated. This indicates that all damage after the first dose must have been repaired, for if it were not, the second dose survival curve would be different, most likely by having a smaller shoulder or perhaps no shoulder.

It is important to emphasize that all of the above discussion regarding repair of sublethal damage applies only to x- or γ-rays. Repair of sublethal damage is practically nonexistent for neutrons.

Sublethal damage and its repair have been measured for almost every cell that can be grown in vitro, and for every normal tissue in

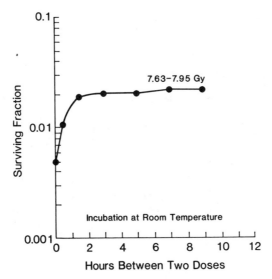

FIG 3–6.
The effect of two doses of radiation separated by various periods of time on surviving fraction in Chinese hamster cells in vitro. The data show that survival is increased if sufficient time is allowed to elapse between two doses of radiation. The increase in survival is due to the repair of sublethal damage. (Redrawn from Elkind MM et al: Radiation response in mammalian cells in culture. V. Temperature dependence of the repair of x-ray damage in surviving cells (aerobic and hypoxic). *Radiat Res* 1965; 25:359–376.)

vivo for which a quantitative endpoint is available. In general, the amount of sublethal damage repair agrees well with the size of the shoulder on the survival curve. Cells and tissues with a broad shoulder on the plotted curve, such as jejunum, exhibit a large amount of sublethal damage repair. Other cells and tissues, such as bone marrow stem cells, have a narrow shoulder on the curve and exhibit little repair of sublethal damage. In terms of the linear quadratic model, cells with a narrow shoulder on the survival curve have a large α/β ratio, whereas cells and tissues with a large shoulder have a small α/β ratio.

The half-time for repair of sublethal damage has been shown consistently to be about 1 hour for cells in vitro, regardless of cell line. However, repair half-times for in vivo systems, specifically normal tissues, have been shown to vary from 0.5 hour to 1.5 hours.

The basis for and the lesions that cause sublethal damage and its repair are unknown. Since the critical target in the cell for radiation is most likely genomic DNA, it is probable that DNA strand breaks are responsible. However, the exact DNA lesion responsible for sublethal damage is unknown.

Sublethal damage and its repair are very important factors in the sparing effect in normal tissues during fractionated radiotherapy. This is discussed in detail in Chapter 10.

Potentially Lethal Damage (PLD)

Even more of an operational term than sublethal damage is potentially lethal damage. This term is quite appropriate, however, since it reflects exactly what is observed. An example may best demonstrate this phenomenon: when cells are placed in suboptimal growth conditions (depleted nutrients) after irradiation, survival is *increased* relative to when these same irradiated cells are incubated in full-growth conditions (nutritionally complete). This damage then has the *potential* to develop, but only if the postirradiation conditions are conducive.

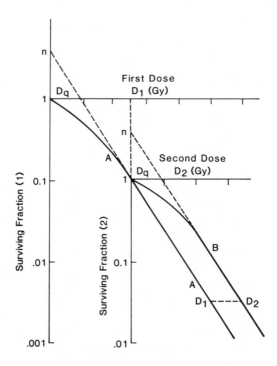

FIG 3–7.
Split-dose survival curves showing the effect of repair of sublethal damage on survival. If sublethal damage is fully repaired, then the slope of the second-dose survival curve (survival curve *B, D₂*) is the same as that for the single-dose survival curve (survival curve *A, D₁*). Note that both the *D_q* and extrapolation number are exactly the same in surviving cells. The first dose has killed a proportion of cells, but surviving cells respond as if they had never been previously irradiated—they have repaired all of their sublethal damage. (Redrawn from Fletcher GH (ed): *Textbook of Radiotherapy,* ed 3. Philadelphia, Lea & Febiger, 1980, p 112.)

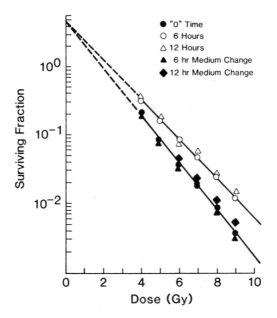

FIG 3–8.
The effect of changing postirradiation conditions on survival of cells in vitro. The *upper curve* represents cells that were not supplied with fresh medium after radiation. The *lower curve* represents cells that were given fresh medium up to 12 hours after radiation. Allowing the cells to remain in the medium in which they were irradiated increases survival, showing that potentially lethal damage can be repaired if the cells are not forced to divide immediately after irradiation. (Redrawn from Little JB: Repair of potentially-lethal radiation damage in mammalian cells: Enhancement by conditioned medium from stationary cultures. *Int J Radiat Biol* 1971; 20:87–92.)

Although this may seem paradoxical (why should a depleted nutritional state *increase* survival, when intuitively one might expect it to *decrease* survival?), placing the cells in suboptimal growth conditions delays their entry into mitosis. Since, in most cases, cell damage is expressed at division, this time permits repair of DNA damage and survival is increased.

This concept was clearly demonstrated by Little, who irradiated cells in conditions suboptimal for cell division, and then either immediately placed the cells into an environment in which they could divide by subculturing them, or kept them under suboptimal conditions for 6 to 12 hours before subculturing them. Survival was increased in cells that remained in the suboptimal growth conditions, compared with cells that were placed in optimal growth conditions, thus being "forced" to divide (Fig 3–8).

Potentially lethal damage and its repair have been demonstrated for cells in culture and in animal tumors, but only after sparsely ionizing radiations. No repair of PLD has been demonstrated after high-LET radiation (e.g., neutrons).

Clearly, an interesting question is whether PLD and SLD are related. Potentially lethal damage differs from SLD in that it is demonstrated after a single dose of radiation, whereas repair of sublethal damage can be demonstrated only after two doses. They appear to be quite different, but the possibility cannot be excluded that they share a common mechanism.

REFERENCES

1. Arena V: *Ionizing Radiations and Life.* St Louis, CV Mosby, 1971.
2. Canti RG, Spear FG: The effect of gamma irradiation on cell division in tissue culture in vitro, Part II. *Proc R Soc Lond [Biol]* 1929; 105:93.
3. Elkind MM, et al: Radiation response in mammalian cells in culture. V. Temperature dependence of the repair of x-ray damage in surviving cells (aerobic and hypoxic). *Radiat Res* 1965; 25:359.
4. Elkind MM, Sutton-Gilbert H: Radiation response of mammalian cells grown in culture. I. Repair of x-ray damage in surviving Chinese hamster cells. *Radiat Res* 1960; 13:556.
5. Kerr FR Jr, Searle J: Apoptosis: Its nature and kinetic role, in Meyn RE, Withers HR (eds): *Radiation Biology in Cancer Research.* New York, Raven Press, 1980, pp 367–384.
6. Kellerer AM, Rosso HH: The theory of dual radiation action. *Curr Topics Radiat Res Q* 1972; 8:85–158.
7. Lea DE: *Actions of Radiations on Living Cells,* ed 2. Cambridge, Cambridge University Press, 1962.
8. Littbrand B, Revesz L: Effects of a second exposure to x-rays on post-irradiation recovery. *Nature* 1967; 214:841.
9. Little JB: Factors influencing the repair of potentially lethal radiation damage in growth-inhibited human cells. *Radiat Res* 1973; 56:320–333.
10. McCulloch EA, Till JE: The sensitivity of cells from normal mouse bone marrow to gamma radiation in vitro and in vivo. *Radiat Res* 1962; 16:822.
11. Puck TT, Marcus TI: Action of x-rays on mammalian cells. *J Exp Med* 1956; 103:653.
12. Withers HR: Recovery and repopulation in vivo by mouse skin epithelial cells during fractionated irradiation. *Radiat Res* 1967; 32:227.
13. Withers HR, Elkind MM: Microcolony survival assay for cells of mouse intestinal mucosa exposed to radiation. *Int J Radiat Biol* 1970; 17:261–267.

Chapter 4 _____

Tissue Radiation Biology

_____

Tissues and organs are made up of cells—in some cases just a few cell types, in other cases many cell types. The underlying assumption throughout this chapter is that the visible and detectable changes induced by radiation, whether at the tissue level or the whole-body level, are due to the killing and subsequent depletion of critical "target" cells in that tissue. In some tissues and organs this target cell has been identified and can be quantified; in others it remains elusive and often controversial despite the efforts of many investigators to identify it. Nonetheless, it is assumed that it is the depletion of these target cells that results in the types of damage to be discussed in this chapter, as well as in Chapters 6 and 7.

Keeping this basic premise in mind, the response of an organ or tissue to radiation depends on two factors:

1. The inherent sensitivity of the various cell populations in that tissue or organ.
2. The turnover kinetics of each population in the tissue (Do they divide, and if so, how often?).

Inherent sensitivity as defined by the loss of reproductive capacity for all cells is similar both in vivo and in vitro (see Chapter 3), yet normal tissues differ widely in their responses to radiation. Thus it must be the "when" and "if" individual cells divide that account for the apparent differences in tissue radiation response. Before tissue response to radiation can be discussed it is necessary to understand the term "sensitivity" and the factors that govern both the sensitivity of individual cells to radiation and the expression of damage following irradiation.

CELLULAR "RADIOSENSITIVITY"

The role of cell division in the radiation response of tissues and organs was appreciated as early as 1906 by two scientists, Bergonié and Tribondeau. Based on physicians' reports that (1) x-rays appeared to destroy the cells of a malignant neoplasm (tumor) without permanently harming the adjacent healthy tissue, and (2) some tissues were damaged by doses of radiation that did not appear to harm other tissues, Bergonié and Tribondeau deduced that cell division was critical to this "selective" cell killing. They performed experiments on rodent testicles to further define this observed selective effect of radiation. They chose the testes because they contain mature cells (spermatozoa), which perform the primary function of the organ, and also contain immature cells (spermatogonia and spermatocytes), which have no function other than to develop into mature, functional cells. Not only do these different populations of cells in the testes vary in function, but their mitotic activity also varies—the immature spermatogonia divide often, whereas the mature spermatogonia never divide.

After irradiation of the testes, Bergonié and Tribondeau observed that the immature dividing cells were damaged after lower doses than were the mature nondividing cells. Based on these observations of the response of the different cell populations in the testes, they formulated a hypothesis concerning radiation sensitivity for all cells in the body. In general terms, their hypothesis states that ionizing radiation is more effective against cells that are actively dividing, are undifferentiated, and have a long dividing future.

Bergonié and Tribondeau defined cell sensitivity in terms of specific cellular characteristics of the cells studied, mitotic activity and differentiation rather than on the radiation. Bergonié and Tribondeau's criteria for cellular radiation sensitivity can be interpreted as determinants of the inherent susceptibility of a cell to radiation damage.

In 1925 Ancel and Vitemberger modified the hypothesis of Bergonié and Tribondeau by proposing that the inherent susceptibility of any cell to damage by ionizing radiation is the same, but that the *time of appearance* of radiation-induced damage differs among different types of cells. In a series of extensive experiments in mammalian systems, they concluded that the appearance of radiation damage is influenced by two factors: (1) the biologic stress on the cell, and (2) the conditions to which the cell is exposed pre-irradiation and postirradiation. On this latter point, Ancel and Vitemberger were well ahead of their time in their thinking, for now, more than 50 years later, it is well known that postirradation conditions can and do affect cellular sensitivity by allowing the expression (or repair) of potentially lethal damage (see Chapter 3).

Ancel and Vitemberger postulated that the greatest influence on radiosensitivity is the biologic stress placed on the cell, and that the most important biologic stress on the cell is the necessity for division. In their terms, all cells will be damaged to the same degree by a given dose of radiation (i.e., all cells are similar in their inherent susceptibility), as has been shown, but the damage will be expressed only *if* and *when* the cell divides. Ancel and Vitemberger were truly clever in their thinking, for they recognized that if all cells had a common target for radiation, then a given dose would deposit the same amount of energy and produce the same amount of damage irrespective of the mitotic status of the cell. However, cells which divided quickly would simply express the damage sooner and appear "sensitive" compared with those that divided more slowly, and would express their damage later and thus appear "resistant."

Thus, in the early twentieth century it was suggested that it was not only cell division and cell turnover that were important in the expression of radiation injury, but also the kinetics of turnover, i.e., whether it occurred rapidly or slowly.

Differentiation

One term that may need clarification is *differentiation*. A differentiated cell is one that is specialized functionally and/or morphologically (structurally); it can be considered a mature cell, or end cell, in a population. An undifferentiated cell has few specialized morphologic or functional characteristics; it is an immature cell whose primary function is to divide, thus providing cells to maintain its own population and to replace mature cells lost from the end cell population. Undifferentiated cells can be considered precursor, or stem, cells in a population.

An example of a tissue that contains a series of cells in various stages of differentiation is the testis. The spermatozoon is the mature, nondividing cell that is morphologically and functionally specialized. However, since mature sperm are periodically lost, more cells must replace them. These cells, also present in the testis, are immature type A spermatogonia; their principal function is to divide and supply the cells that will mature into spermatozoa. The spermatozoan is a differentiated cell; it is the end cell in the population. The spermatogonium is an undifferentiated cell—the stem cell for the mature spermatozoan. The process by which immature spermatogonia become mature spermatozoa is termed differentiation (Fig 4–1).

Another example of a differentiated cell is the erythrocyte (red blood cell, or RBC). Just as the spermatozoan is the mature end cell in the testis, the RBC is the mature, differentiated cell in the red cell line of the hemopoietic system. The major function of the RBC is to transport oxygen to cells of the body. Not only is this cell specialized in function, but it also is specialized in structure; the RBC differs from other cells in the body in that it does not have a nucleus. Therefore, both morphologically and functionally, RBCs are differentiated cells. The average lifetime of RBCs in the circulating blood is 120 days, necessitating a continual replacement of these cells by newly produced cells. The *stem cell* (see below) for the RBC, the erythroblast, is present in the bone marrow and is an undifferentiated cell that divides and supplies cells which will differentiate to become erythrocytes.

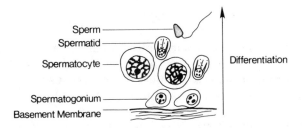

FIG 4–1.
Diagrammatic representation of the testes illustrating differentiation. The cell becomes more differentiated as it progresses from spermatogonium (stem cell) to sperm (end cell).

CELL POPULATIONS

For our purposes here, cell populations can be divided into three categories:

1. Stem cell population
2. Transit cell population
3. Static population

A *stem cell population* is one whose sole purpose is to divide to (1) first maintain its own population (i.e., self-renewal), and (2) produce cells for another population. Stem cells are undifferentiated. Classic examples of stem cell populations are basal cells in the epidermis of the skin, cells in the bone marrow, the cells in the crypts of Lieberkühn in the intestine, and spermatogonia in the testis. Tissues and organs containing stem cell populations are referred to as self-renewing.

Transit cell populations are defined precisely by their name—they are cells on their way from one place (stem cell compartment) to another place (end cell compartment). While in transit these cells may or may not divide. An example of a cell that divides while in transit is the nucleated red cell. A cell that does not divide is the reticulocyte in the bone marrow; it simply receives precursor cells and sends them on their way into the peripheral blood.

The third population, a *static population*, loses cells throughout the life of the organism. These cells are fully differentiated and exhibit no, or at least little, detectable mitotic activity. Examples of such populations are found in adult nervous tissue and muscle.

RADIATION RESPONSE OF CELLS

Based on the aforementioned cell population categories, Rubin and Casarett have defined five categories of cell populations (Table 4–1) in terms of their radiation sensitivities. The criteria used were histologic signs of cell death, not the loss of proliferative potential.

Vegetative Intermitotic Cells (VIM).—VIM cells are rapidly dividing, undifferentiated cells that have a short lifetime. According to Bergonié and Tribondeau, these cells comprise the most radiation-sensitive group of cells in the body. Examples of VIM cells are basal cells of the epidermis, crypt cells of the intestines, type A spermatogonia, and erythroblasts.

Differentiating Intermitotic Cells (DIM).—DIM cells are produced by division of VIM cells and, although actively mitotic, they are more differentiated than VIM cells. Therefore, these cells are less sensitive (or more resistant) to radiation than are the VIM cells. Examples of DIM cells are intermediate and type B spermatogonia.

Multipotential Connective Tissue Cells.—These cells divide irregularly, are more differentiated than either VIM or DIM cells, and are intermediate in sensitivity to radiation. Cells included in this category are endothelial cells (blood vessel liners) and fibroblasts (composing connective tissue).

Reverting Postmitotic Cells (RPM).—Cells in this category normally do not undergo mitosis; however, they retain the capability of division under specific circumstances. RPM cells are long-lived as individuals and are more differentiated than cells of the previous categories; therefore, RPM cells are relatively radioresistant. Examples of RPM cells are liver cells and the mature lymphocyte. The mature lymphocyte is included in this category because of its mitotic characteristics—it does not usually divide, but has the capability of dividing when a stimulus is present. The lymphocyte also is a differentiated cell; however, in contrast to other RPM cells that are relatively radioresistant, the mature lymphocyte is very radiosensitive. It is one important exception to the general law of Bergonié and Tribondeau.

Fixed Postmitotic Cells (FPM).—FPM cells do not divide. These cells are highly differentiated both morphologically and functionally; therefore, they are resistant to radiation. In fact, this category comprises

TABLE 4–1.

Characteristics and Radiosensitivities of Mammalian Cell Populations

Cell Type	Characteristics	Examples	Radiosensitivity
VIM	Divide regularly and rapidly; undifferentiated; do not differentiate between divisions	Type A spermatogonia, erythroblasts, crypt cells of intestines, basal cells of epidermis	High
DIM	Actively dividing; more differentiated than VIMs; differentiate between divisions	Intermediate spermatogonia, myelocytes	
Multipotential connective tissue	Irregularly dividing; more differentiated than VIMs or DIMs	Endothelial cells, fibroblasts	
RPM	Do not normally divide, but retain capability of division; variably differentiated	Parenchymal cells of liver, lymphocytes*	
FPM	Do not divide; highly differentiated	Nerve cells, muscle cells, erythrocytes (RBCs), spermatozoa	Low

*Lymphocytes, although classified as relatively radioresistant by their characteristics, are very radiosensitive.

TABLE 4–2.

Cell Classification by Decreasing Radiosensitivity*

Group	Sensitivity	Examples
1	High	Mature lymphocytes, erythroblasts, certain spermatogonia
2		Granulosa cells, myelocytes, intestinal crypt cells, basal cells of epidermis
3		Endothelial cells, gastric gland cells, osteoblasts, chondroblasts, spermatocytes, spermatids
4		Granulocytes, osteocytes, spermatozoa, erythrocytes
5	Low	Fibrocytes, chondrocytes, muscle cells, nerve cells

*From Casarett AP: *Radiation Biology.* Englewood Cliffs, NJ, Prentice-Hall, 1968. Used by permission.

the group of cells most resistant to radiation. Some of the cells in this category have long lives, whereas others are relatively short-lived. When the short-lived cells die, they are replaced by differentiating (DIM) cells. Other cells in this category may not be replaced if cell death occurs. Examples of cells in this category include some nerve cells, muscle cells, erythrocytes (RBCs), and spermatozoa.

Table 4–2 gives a classification of cells according to decreasing radiosensitivity, again using histologic signs of cell death as the determining factor.

TISSUE RESPONSE TO RADIATION

It was pointed out in Chapter 3 that the D_o for mammalian cells obtained both in vivo and in vitro is between 1 and 2 Gy, indicating that there is not a substantial difference in the radiosensitivity of mammalian cells. However, it is well known that there is a vast difference in the doses at which different organs and tissues exhibit damage. Reasons for these dose differences must be sought elsewhere. Since cell division is necessary for radiation damage to be expressed, then the time of expression of injury in an organ must be dependent on the turnover time of the critical target cells—not only if they divide, but when and how often. The term target cell does not imply that radiation is selective for any given cell, but refers to those cells in the tissue that can divide and regenerate the tissue after radiation, i.e., the stem cells. When sufficient numbers of cells are killed and subsequently depleted due to a failure of the stem cells to regenerate after irradiation, overt functional and structural tissue damage occurs. Thus, to understand tissue response to radiation it is important to first have some knowledge of how tissues and organs are organized. This knowledge also is critical to an understanding of how the effects of radiation on different tissues are measured.

Tissue Organization

Tissues and organs are made up of two compartments: the parenchymal compartment, containing the cells characteristic of that individual tissue or organ, and the stromal compartment, composed of connective tissue and vasculature, which makes up the supporting structure of the organ (Fig 4–2).

The parenchymal compartment of tissues and organs may be composed of one or more than one category of cells, as defined by Rubin and Casarett. The testis is an example of an organ that contains more than one category of cells: stem cells—type A spermatogonia (VIM cells); intermediate cells—type B spermatogonia, spermatocytes, and spermatids (DIM cells); and mature, functional cells—spermatozoa (FPM cells). Another example is the hemopoietic system: the bone marrow contains the undifferentiated stem cells, and the circulating blood contains the mature end cell. Two other examples are the skin and the intestinal tract.

In these types of organs where the parenchymal compartment is composed of various cellular populations, cells flow from the stem cell compartment to the differentiated compartment to the end cell compartment as needed (Fig 4–3).

Examples of tissues and organs whose parenchymal compartments

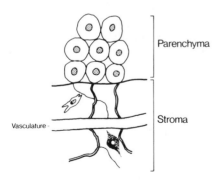

FIG 4–2.
Diagram of the parenchymal and stromal compartments of any organ. The parenchymal compartment contains cells typical of the organ, whereas the stromal compartment contains connective tissue, *(light-colored background),* vasculature and other cells such as mast cells *(below vessel)* and fibrocytes *(above vessel).*

FIG 4–3.
Flow of the cell from the stem cell compartment *(VIM)* to differentiating compartment *(DIM)* to the end cell compartment *(FPM),* illustrated by cells of the testis.

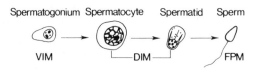

are composed of only RPM cells or FPM cells are the liver, muscle, brain, and spinal cord. The hepatic cells of the liver are RPM cells, dividing only when the need exists. If a partial hepatectomy is performed, the hepatic cells will begin to divide and replace the part of the liver that has been removed. However, most cells of the brain and most muscle cells do not retain the capability of division; these tissues and organs are composed of FPM cells.

Regardless of the population of cells in the parenchymal compartment, all tissues and organs will have a supporting stromal compartment composed of connective tissue and vasculature (multipotential connective tissue cells).

Mechanisms of Damage in Normal Tissues

Tables 4–1 and 4–2 indicate that cells in the vasculature are intermediate in sensitivity to radiation, i.e., they are more sensitive than either the RPM or FPM cells of organs such as the lung, kidney, and spinal cord. For this reason, it had long been suggested that damage in such tissues was a consequence of damage to the vasculature (tissue damage occurred indirectly via vascular narrowing and occlusion, resulting in tissue ischemia), rather than damage to cells specific to that organ (the parenchyma). Recently, however, this hypothesis has been questioned and, in fact, a new classification of normal tissue responses according to the time in which the tissues express injury has been suggested. This new hypothesis states that the response in all normal tissues is due to killing and subsequent depletion of the critical parenchymal cells of that organ, and that the differences in the time it takes for damage to be expressed are due simply to differences in turnover kinetics of the target cells. The current philosophy, then, is that tissue damage is due to depletion of critical target cells and is not an indirect result of vascular damage. For example, damage is seen in the intestine within a week to 10 days after irradiation, and is quite predictable based on the turnover kinetics of the stem cells in the crypts (i.e., 12-hour cell cycle). On the other hand, damage in the lung is not expressed for at least 3 months after irradiation, which, rather than being a consequence of vascular damage, most likely reflects the slow turnover of the critical parenchymal cells in the lung (perhaps type 2 cells), whose loss results in observable damage.

Based on the difference in turnover kinetics of the critical target cells in different tissues, normal tissues can be divided into two categories: acutely responding and late responding normal tissues. The acutely responding tissues manifest their injury within a few months after radiation is completed because they are self-renewal tissues containing rapidly dividing stem cell populations. Examples are the bone marrow, skin, intestine, and testis. On the other hand, late responding normal tissues do not express injury for at least 3 months or longer because they contain slowly dividing cell populations. Two examples of the latter are lung and kidney.

Thus, differences in the times within which different tissues express damage after radiation are most likely not an issue of vascular vs. parenchyma, but rather are due simply to the fact that some cells in some tissues, such as the lung, divide more slowly than cells in other tissues, such as the intestine. Table 4–3 lists acutely responding and late responding normal tissues and the known or hypothesized critical target cells.

TABLE 4–3.

Acutely Responding and Late Responding Normal Tissues

Tissue	Target Cells
Acutely responding	
Skin	Basal cells of the epidermis
Hair	Follicle
Lip mucosa	Basal cells
Jejunum	Crypt cells
Colon	Crypt cells
Testis	Spermatogonia
Bone marrow	Stem cells
Late responding	
Kidney	? Epithelial cells of proximal tubules
Lung	? Type 2 pneumonocytes
Spinal cord	Glial cell
Brain	?
Bladder	?

MEASUREMENT OF RADIATION DAMAGE IN TISSUES

Assays of Tissue Response

In order to compare and contrast the responses of different tissues to radiation, assays that allow the assessment of damage as a function of dose are essential. Two criteria are necessary for an assay of tissue effect to be of value:

1. It must be quantifiable (i.e., assign a number to it).
2. The effect must increase with increasing radiation dose.

Many techniques that meet these criteria for a wide variety of normal tissue are now available for measuring tissue response to radiation in experimental animals. These techniques either provide cell survival curves or dose response curves.

There are many ways to assess the effects of radiation on tissues in vivo, but for our purposes the most critical test will be the ability of the dividing clonogenic (stem) cells to undergo unlimited division, i.e., to retain their reproductive integrity. It is clear that such an assay is reasonable for cells grown in vitro. In this situation cell survival can be assessed as a function of dose and cell survival curves obtained. The questions are whether it is possible to obtain survival curves for cells of tissues in vivo and, if it is not, how tissue responses to radiation are then measured.

Assays of damage in organized tissues and organs can be divided into three categories:

1. Clonogenic (related to the reproductive integrity of the clonogenic stem cells in the tissue)
2. Specific tissue function
3. Lethality

Clonogenic Assays

Based on the previous discussion of cell populations, it is clear that if a tissue contains stem cells that divide and form clones in vivo, and if these stem cells can be easily identified and quantified, then the construction of survival curves for the target cells of this tissue in situ is possible. There are a number of such "clonogenic" assays for some normal tissues: bone marrow, testis, and mammary and thyroid glands, to name just a few. In some of these, clonogenic survival is assessed in situ in the same animal that was previously irradiated (skin, basal cells of the epidermis; intestine, number of surviving crypt cells; testis, number of tubules containing spermatogenic epithelium). In others, the cells are taken from the irradiated animal (donor) and transplanted into a genetically identical mouse for assay.

In Situ Assays.—Withers and his colleagues have been instrumental in developing in situ clonogenic assays for a number of normal tissues, including skin, intestine, testis, and kidney. The intestine will be used to illustrate this technique.

The intestine is an example of a tissue in which dividing cells are confined to one location, the crypts of Lieberkühn. These cells divide about every 12 hours, replacing their own population, plus providing a constant supply of cells for the nondividing differentiated cells that are sloughed from the villi every 24 hours. The villi are dependent on the crypts for cell replacement; if the cells in the crypt are dead, the villi become shortened, flattened, and partially or completely denuded. In the intestine, then, damage is due to killing, with subsequent depletion of the cells in the crypts of Lieberkühn followed by denudation of the epithelial lining of the mucosa. Figure 4–4 shows a control, nonirradiated intestine tissue (A), and two examples of irradiated intestine tissue (B and C). Because the crypts are easily identified using the light microscope, the number of surviving crypts can be counted and plotted as a function of dose. Since it is assumed that a crypt can be repopulated by one surviving cell, a cell survival curve can be constructed. An example of such a crypt cell survival curve is given in Figure 4–5. Similar techniques are used in the testis and skin to obtain cell survival curves. In all of these acutely responding normal tissues, survival is assayed within a month after irradiation, reflecting the rapid turnover of the clonogenic stem cells in each tissue.

Recently, Withers and his colleagues have developed an in situ clonogenic assay for kidney, a late responding normal tissue. The underlying hypothesis on which the assay is based is that radiation damage in the kidney is due to depletion of the parenchymal cells, specifically the epithelial cells of the proximal tubules.

At first glance this may seem surprising, since the cells of the tubule epithelium are well differentiated and divide very slowly. However, unlike the other tissues in which damage is expressed within a month after irradiation (3 days in intestine, 2 to 3 weeks in skin, and 4 weeks in the testis), damage in the kidney is expressed at 1 year after irradiation, reflecting the slow turnover of the tubule cells suggested to be the critical cells killed by radiation. The survival curve for epithelial cells in kidney tubule is shown in Figure 4–6. The D_0 for these cells is 1.5 Gy. Thus, the target cells for this late responding normal tissue have sensitivity similar to that of the acutely responding normal tissues.

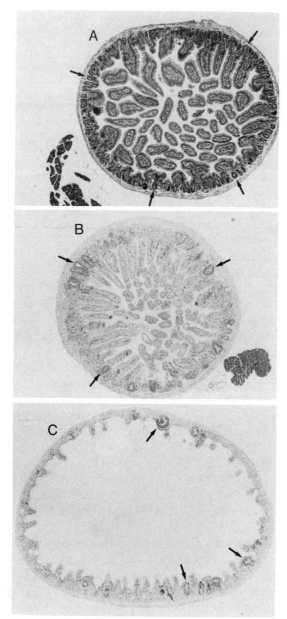

FIG 4–4.
Examples of jejunal tissue from (**A**) a nonirradiated mouse, (**B**) a mouse given a moderate single dose of radiation, and (**C**) a mouse given a high single dose of radiation. Crypts are easily recognizable *(arrows).* They are quantifiable, and cell survival curves can be constructed from the data. (Magnification × 100.)

Transplantation Assays.—The assays of clonogenic survival in bone marrow and thyroid and mammary glands require that the irradiated tissue be removed from the animal and a single cell suspension be made and then injected into another animal. In other words, the recipient animal acts like a culture dish. This technique is best illustrated by the bone marrow colony-forming units (CFUs) assay developed by Till and McCulloch: (1) animals are irradiated to the whole body with a range of doses, (2) bone marrow is removed from their legs, and (3) single cell suspensions are made, various amounts of which are injected into previously irradiated syngeneic recipient animals. (The recipient animals must be previously irradiated so that all their bone marrow cells are destroyed, allowing the cells of the donor mice to grow.) These donor cells colonize the bone marrow and spleen, forming visible colonies in the latter. The spleen is removed 9 days later and the number

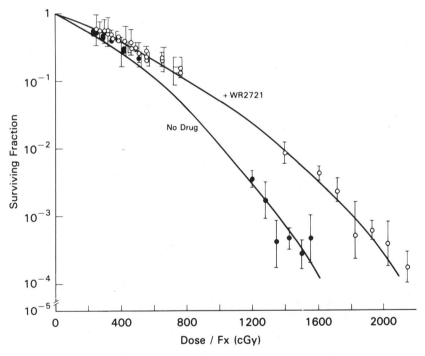

FIG 4–5.
Survival of crypt cells following radiation either alone or in the presence of a known radioprotector, WR-2721. (Redrawn from Travis EL et al, Protection of mouse jejunal crypt cells by WR-2721 after small doses of radiation. *Int J Radiat Oncol Biol Phys* 1986; 12:807–814.) (FX = fraction.)

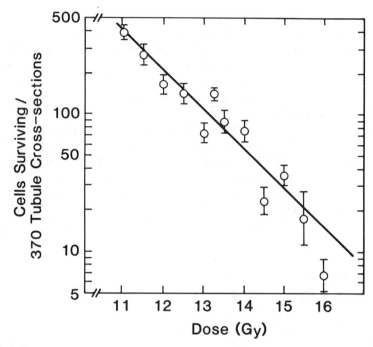

FIG 4–6.
Dose survival curves for kidney tubule cells showing a D_o of about 1.5 Gy. (From Withers HR, Mason KA, Thames HD Jr: *Br J Radiol* 1986; 59:587–595. Used by permission.)

of colonies counted, each of which is assumed to have arisen from the injection of one surviving cell. The number of colonies after each dose is counted, the proportion of cells surviving calculated and plotted as a function of dose. An example of a survival curve for bone marrow cells is given in Figure 4–7. Similar assays are available for thyroid and mammary glands.

Survival curves for all clonogenic assays in vivo are plotted in Figure 4–8. Although there is a range of sensitivities, the biggest difference between these survival curves for tissues is the shoulder, not the slope (i.e., D_o values are more similar than the shoulders). Although the data for the kidney are not plotted, it is clear that the kidney has a similar sensitivity to the more rapidly dividing normal tissues, i.e., the D_o is within the range for the rapidly dividing normal tissues.

Functional Assays

Many tissues do not have clonogenic stem cells that can be readily identified and quantified, particularly those tissues classified as late responding. Thus our knowledge of how these tissues respond to radiation has been minimal. However, it is obvious that these tissues are as important as the acutely responding normal tissues for obtaining a favorable outcome when treating a tumor with radiation. This has prompted the development of new assays of function for many tissues. These functional endpoints meet the criteria that damage must increase as a function of dose. Such data produce dose response curves rather than cell survival curves, and although they tell little about the survival of the underlying putative target cells, they do allow comparison of tissue responses to radiation. Most of these are based on either the

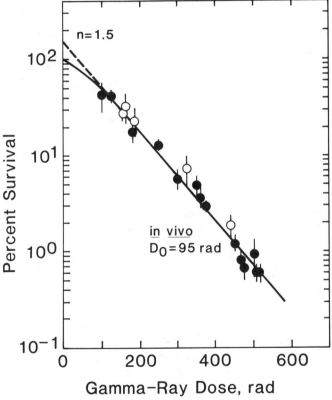

FIG 4–7.
Percent survival as a function of dose for colony-forming ability of mouse bone marrow cells. This is an example of a survival curve from a transplantation assay. The cells are irradiated in a donor and then transferred to a lethally irradiated recipient, and the resultant spleen colonies are counted. (Redrawn from McCullough EA, Till JE: The sensitivity of cells from normal mouse bone marrow to gamma radiation in vitro and in vivo. *Radiat Res* 1962; 16:822–832.)

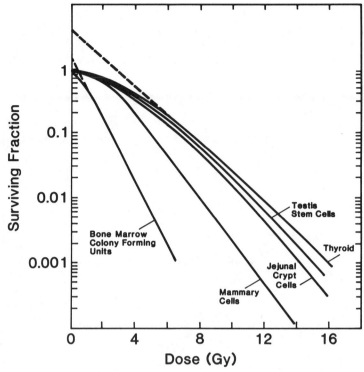

FIG 4–8.
Survival curves as a function of dose for a number of clonogenic assays in vivo, showing that the slopes of the survival curves are similar (D_o values fall within a narrow range). However, the biggest variation in these survival curves is in the shoulder region. (Redrawn from Hall EJ: *Radiobiology for the Radiologist,* ed 3. Philadelphia, JB Lippincott, 1988, p 56. Used by permission.)

physiology of the organ (e.g., breathing rate measurements after lung irradiation, frequency of urination after bladder irradiation), whereas others rely on scoring visible changes in the organ that occur after irradiation (e.g., acute skin reactions consisting of hair loss, erythema, and desquamation). Such techniques have been invaluable in increasing our understanding of the responses of late responding normal tissues to radiation.

Lethality
The single most often used nonclonogenic assay for quantifying damage in normal tissues is lethality. In these studies the number of animals dead after localized irradiation of a *specific organ* is quantified as a function of dose and dose response curves are then constructed.

The lethal dose that kills 50% of the animals, LD_{50} is obtained for different normal tissues, allowing comparisons of the dose for this same effect (called isoeffect) between tissues.

The LD_{50} for a given tissue is further defined by the time when deaths occur. Based on the assumption that cell division is necessary for radiation damage to be expressed, deaths would occur quickly after irradiation of the intestine (by irradiating the whole abdomen), but much more slowly after irradiation of the lungs, reflecting the differences in turnover times of the critical cells in these two tissues.

Figure 4–9 presents a series of dose response curves for lethality after localized irradiation of different normal tissues. For comparison, the dose response curve for spinal cord paralysis is also shown. The LD_{50} for each tissue is given in Table 4–4.

Table 4–5 lists all the quantitative endpoints which are available for assessing the response of normal tissues to radiation in experimental animals.

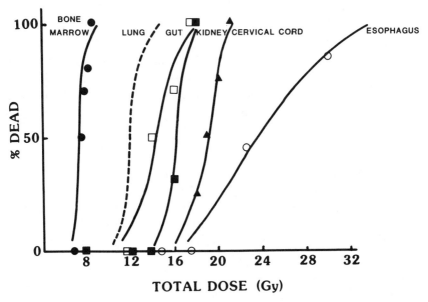

FIG 4–9.
Number of animals dead is a function of dose for six different normal tissues. In general, the curves are very steep, although they are displaced on the dose axis, bone marrow being most "sensitive," and esophagus, most "resistant." (Redrawn from Travis EL: *Relative radiosensitivity of the human being. Adv Radiat Biol* 1987; 12:205–238.)

TABLE 4–4.

LD_{50} Values Estimated From Dose-Response Curves for Radiation Damage to Various Normal Tissues in Experimental Animals

Tissue	Animal	Assay	LD_{50} (Gy)
Bone marrow	Mouse	Death, 30 days	7.20
Lung	Mouse	Death, 80–100 days	12.34
Gut*	Mouse	Death, 10–12 days	14.20
Kidney	Mouse	Death, 500 days	16.00
Spinal cord[†]	Rat	Paralysis, 7 mos	19.00
Esophagus	Mouse	Death, 20 days	24.80

*Total abdominal irradiation.
[†]ED_{50} effect dose 50; used in tissues where an effect other than death is quantified; for example, paralysis after spinal cord irradiation.

SHAPES OF SURVIVAL CURVES FOR ACUTELY RESPONDING AND LATE RESPONDING NORMAL TISSUES

It is now possible to construct dose survival curves for many normal tissues in vivo. However, for those tissues for which clonogenic assays do not exist because the target cells in the tissue are either unknown or cannot be quantitatively assessed, survival curves can only be deduced from their dose response curves. Based on such deductions, it has been suggested that not only do acutely and late responding normal tissues express their damage at vastly different times, but that their survival curves for the "target" cells are also different. Shown in Figure 4–10 are dose survival curves for an acutely responding and a late responding normal tissue. It is clear that the shapes of the survival curves for the two classes of tissue differ, and that the curve for late responding normal tissues is "curvier" than that for acutely responding normal tissues. Some knowledge of the differences in survival curve shapes is important to an understanding of the factors that govern cellular and tissue responses, since modifiers of radiation damage may differentially affect these two classes of normal tissues. This hypothesis has important implications for dose fractionation as used in radiotherapy and is fully discussed in Chapter 10.

TABLE 4–5.
Quantitative Normal Tissue Endpoints

Tissue	Clonogenic	Functional	Lethality
Bone marrow	Spleen colonies (transplantation)		$LD_{50/30 \text{ days}}$
Intestine	Crypt colonies (in situ)		$LD_{50/7-10 \text{ days}}$
Testis	Tubules with spermatogonic epithelium (in situ)	Weight	—
Skin	Skin colonies (in situ)	Early skin reaction, late deformities	—
Esophagus	—		$LD_{50/28-60 \text{ days}}$
Mammary gland	Transplantation		—
Liver	In situ		—
Thyroid	Transplantation		—
Kidney	Tubules with epithelial cells	^{51}Cr EDTA clearance, hematocrit, urination frequency, weight	$LD_{50/12-15 \text{ mos}}$
Lung	—	Breathing rate, CO_2 clearance	$LD_{50/80-180 \text{ days}}$ $LD_{50/360 \text{ days}}$
Bladder		Urination frequency, contracture	—
CNS	—		Incidence of paralysis, $ED_{50/7 \text{ mos}}$, $ED_{50/18 \text{ mos}}$

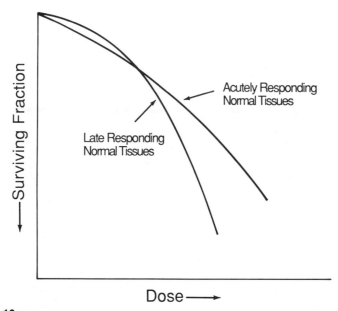

FIG 4–10.
Schematic of the hypothesized survival curves for acutely responding and late responding normal tissues. The curve for the late responding normal tissues is "curvier" than that for the acutely responding normal tissues.

REFERENCES

1. Ancel P, Vitemberger P: Sur la radiosensibilite cellulaire. *C R Soc Biol* 1925; 92:517.
2. Bergonié J, Tribondeau L: De quelques resultats de la radiotherapie et essai de fixation d'une technique rationelle. *C R Acad Sci (Paris)* 1906; 143:983.
3. Casarett AP: *Radiation Biology.* Englewood Cliffs, NJ, Prentice-Hall, 1968.
4. DeMott RK, Mulcahy RT, Clifton KH: The survival of thyroid cells following irradiation: A directly generated single-dose survival curve. *Radiat Res* 1979; 77:395–403.
5. Fowler JF, Morgan RL, Silvester JA, et al: Experiments with fractionated x-ray treatment of the skin of pigs. I. Fractionation up to 28 days. *Br J Radiol* 1963; 36:188–196.
6. Gilbert CW, Lajtha LG: The importance of cell population kinetics in determining response to irradiation of normal and malignant tissues, in *Cellular Radiation Biology,* Eighteenth Annual Symposium on Fundamental Cancer Research, The University of Texas M D Anderson Hospital and Tumor Institute. Baltimore, Williams & Wilkins, 1965.

7. Gould MN, Clifton KH: The survival of mammary cells following irradiation *in vivo*: a directly generated single-dose survival curve. *Radiat Res* 1977; 72:343–352.

8. Rubin P, Casarett GW: *Clinical Radiation Pathology*, vols I and II. Philadelphia, WB Saunders, 1968.

9. Thames HD, Withers HR, Peters LJ, et al: Changes in early and late radiation responses with altered dose fractionation: Implications for dose-survival relationships. *Int J Radiat Oncol Biol Phys* 1982; 8:219–226.

10. Till JE, McCulloch EA: A direct measurement of the radiation sensitivity of normal mouse bone marrow cells. *Radiat Res* 1961; 14:213–222.

11. Travis EL: Relative radiosensitivity of the human lung. *Adv Radiat Biol* 1987; 12:205–238.

12. Travis EL, Down JD, Holmes SJ, et al: Radiation pneumonitis and fibrosis in mouse lung assayed by respiratory frequency and histology. *Radiat Res* 1980; 84:133–143.

13. Travis EL, Thames HD Jr, Tucker SL, et al: Protection of mouse jejunal crypt cells by WR-2721 after small doses of radiation. *Int J Radiat Oncol Biol Phys* 1986; 12:807–814.

14. Travis EL, Vojnovic B, Davies EE, et al: A plethysmographic method for measuring function in locally irradiated mouse lung. *Br J Radiol* 1979; 52:67–74.

15. Withers HR, Elkind MM: Microcolony survival assay for cells of mouse intestinal mucosa exposed to radiation. *Int J Radiat Biol* 1970; 17:261–267.

16. Withers HR, Hunter N, Barkley HT Jr, Reid BO: Radiation survival and regeneration characteristics of spermatogenic stem cells of mouse testis. *Radiat Res* 1974; 57:88–103.

17. Withers HR, Mason KA, Thames HD Jr: Late radiation response of kidney assayed by tubule cell survival. *Br J Radiol* 1986; 59:587–595.

Modification of Cell and Tissue Responses to Radiation

_____

Physical Factors
  LET and RBE
  Dose Rate
Chemical Factors
  Radiation Sensitizers—Oxygen
  Other Sensitizers
  Radiation Protectors
Biologic Factors
  Cell Cycle
  Intracellular Repair

The response of cells and tissues to radiation can be affected by various factors; the effects are either to diminish the response, enhance the response, or elicit the response at a different time. Therefore, these factors *appear* to affect the radiosensitivity of cells and tissues—cells and tissues exhibiting enhanced response appear more radiosensitive; those exhibiting diminished response appear more radioresistant. However, the inherent sensitivity of the cell has not changed; the cell is basically the same with the same characteristics (i.e., dividing or non-dividing and differentiated or undifferentiated). What has changed is an external factor such as the linear energy transfer (LET) of the radiation or the environment in which the cell is growing, thus exerting an influence on the response of the cell (or organism) to radiation. These factors are those that Ancel and Vitemberger identified as affecting cellular radiosensitivity, factors to which the cell is exposed pre- or post-irradiation.

The factors affecting cell and tissue responses will be discussed in this chapter. They are grouped as *physical factors, chemical factors,* and *biologic factors.*

PHYSICAL FACTORS

LET and RBE

As discussed in Chapter 2, the quality of the radiation has an effect on the biologic response. Linear energy transfer (LET) is the term that describes the rate at which energy is lost from different types of radiation while traveling through matter. Irradiation of the same biologic system with different LET radiations will produce differences in the severity of the same biologic response. The term relating biologic response to the quality of the radiation is *RBE.*

To compare the effect on cell survival of high-LET radiations (e.g., neutrons) to low-LET radiations (e.g., x-rays), survival curves are constructed of cells exposed to these two types of radiation (Fig 5–1). RBE can be calculated from this curve by choosing the same survival level on the exponential portion of both curves—e.g., 0.1, 0.01, or the D_o dose—and comparing the doses from the two types of radiation that produce this response. In the example in Figure 5–1, 10 Gy of x-rays and 6.5 Gy of neutrons produce a surviving fraction of 0.01. Therefore, the RBE of neutrons equals 1.5, which can be interpreted to mean that neutrons are 50% more effective than x-rays in killing 99% of a population of cells.

Figure 5–2 shows survival curves for various types of clonogenic mammalian cells after x- or neutron irradiation. D_o and D_q values are also given in this figure. Although there is a wide range of values for both D_o and D_q for these different normal mammalian cell lines after x-irradiation, the biggest variability is in the size and shape of the initial portion of the survival curves (Fig 5–2). These differences are attributable to differences in the inherent radioresistance of these cells, and are manifested as differences in repair of sublethal damage, generally defined by the size and shape of the shoulder of the survival curve. Neutrons reduce these differences in response between cell types by reducing the size and variability of the shoulder region of the survival curve. Although there is still a range of responses after neutron irradiation, the differences between the various cell types are now much smaller. The reason for these differences is attributable to the way in which neutrons and x-rays deposit their energy. Low-LET radiation (x-rays) produces sparse ionizations separated by relatively long distances,

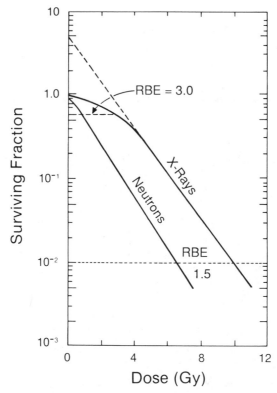

FIG 5–1.
Survival curves for mammalian cells exposed to single doses of x-rays or neutrons. Neutrons have two effects on the x-ray survival curve: (1) they reduce the shoulder and (2) the slope becomes steeper. For this reason the RBE measured after a small dose is higher (3.0) than the RBE measured after a high dose (1.5). (Redrawn from Hall EJ, *Radiobiology for the Radiologist,* ed 3. Philadelphia, JB Lippincott, 1988.)

whereas high-LET radiation produces dense ionizations in very short distances. The ionization density produced by high- and low-LET radiations in the same population of cells is illustrated in Fig 5–3. The high-LET radiation has produced two hits in the nuclei of two different cells, whereas the low-LET radiation has produced only one hit in the nuclei of two cells. If we assume that most mammalian cells contain more than one target that must be hit to cause cell death, and that these targets are contained within the nucleus, it can readily be seen that the high-LET radiation with its high ionization density is more efficient in producing cell death than the low-LET radiation. The decrease or absence of the shoulder region on the survival curve of cells irradiated with high-LET radiations, then, is due to the large number of ionizations produced in the targets.

In some systems (e.g., viruses) a single ionization in the target volume will result in death of the organism. In this type of system many of the ionizations from high-LET radiations will be wasted; if only one hit is required to kill the organism, two hits will not render it "more dead." Therefore, in these systems low-LET radiations will be more efficient for producing cell killing than high-LET radiations on a dose basis.

Because neutrons differentially affect the shoulder of the x-ray survival curve of mammalian cells more than the slope, the RBE will not be a constant factor over the whole dose range and will become *larger*

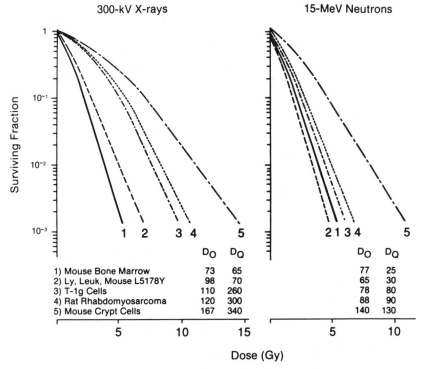

FIG 5–2.
Survival curves for various types of mammalian cells irradiated with 300-kV x-rays or 15-MeV neutrons. The wide variability in both shoulder and slope for x-ray survival curves is less marked after neutron irradiation, i.e., neutrons appear to smooth out the differences in the survival curves of mammalian cells. (From Broerse JJ, Barendsen GW: Current topics. *Radiat Res* 1973; 8:305–350. Used by permission.)

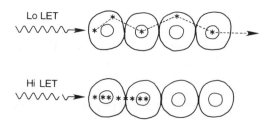

FIG 5–3.

Comparison of the effects of low- and high-LET radiations on a population of cells. Note the irregular path of the low-LET radiation interacting with four cells, compared with the relatively straight path of the high-LET radiation interacting with only two cells. However, the low-LET radiation produces only *one* hit in two nuclei, whereas the high-LET radiation produces *two* hits in two nuclei.

as the dose is reduced. This can be understood by again looking at Figure 5–1, which shows that the x-ray dose at a survival level of 0.6 is 3 Gy, whereas the neutron dose for this same survival level is only 1 Gy; thus the RBE is 3. This has important implications for clinical radiotherapy, which uses small dose fractions in the shoulder region of the curve (see Chapter 10).

Because of their differential effect on the shoulder of the survival curve for mammalian cells, the effectiveness of neutrons in comparison with that of x-rays for both tissue damage or cell kill (RBE) depends on the tissue and the dose per fraction. (RBE is the relative biologic effect, the ratio of dose of x-rays to dose of neutrons producing equivalent biologic damage, as discussed in detail in Chapter 2.) In general, RBE increases as the dose per fraction decreases, but the RBE and dose-per-fraction relationship is critically dependent on the size and shape of the initial portion of the survival curve of the tissue's putative target cells, and thus will vary among tissues. As discussed in Chapter 4, the shapes of the survival curves for the underlying target cells in different tissues are known to vary, some curves having large shoulders, such as intestine, and others, such as bone marrow, having small shoulders. In general, cells and tissues that have large shoulders on the survival curves after x-irradiation will exhibit higher RBEs with neutrons than cells and tissues with small shoulders.

Dose Rate

Another physical factor affecting the response of cells to radiation is dose rate, i.e., the rate at which the radiation is delivered. A dose-rate effect has been observed in many types of biologic damage, including reproductive failure, division delay, chromosome aberrations (especially complex aberrations), and survival times of organisms exposed to total body irradiation. All studies have shown low dose rates to be less efficient for producing damage than high dose rates.

This is clearly shown in Figure 5–4, where an established mammalian cell line (Chinese hamster ovary cells) was irradiated with dose rates ranging from a high of 1.07 Gy/min to a low of 0.0036 Gy/min. Survival clearly increased as the dose rate decreased. The overall effect on the survival curve of reducing the dose rate is that the slope becomes

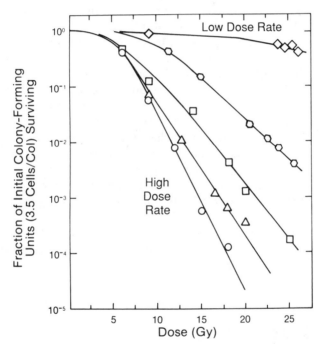

FIG 5–4.
Dose response curves for an established mammalian cell line irradiated with a wide range of dose rates from a high of 1.07 Gy/min to a low of 0.0036 Gy/min. Reducing the dose rate makes the survival curve more shallow and causes the shoulder to disappear. Survival approaches an exponential function of dose as the dose rate is reduced. (From Bedford JS, Mitchell JB: Dose-rate effects in synchronous mammalian cells in culture. *Radiat Res* 1973; 54:316–327. Used by permission.)

more shallow and the shoulder disappears. Essentially, as the dose rate is reduced, survival approaches an exponential function of dose and, in fact, at very low doses will be exponential. The slope of this curve will be the same as that of the *initial portion* of the acute single-dose survival curve and not that of the terminal exponential region. The dose-rate effect is most dramatic between 0.01 and 1 Gy/min (1 to 100 rad/min), and is less marked above and below this dose rate; the survival curve changes little, if at all, in these ranges.

An explanation for the dependence of biologic response on dose rate is that low dose rates allow repair to occur before enough damage has accumulated to cause death of the cell. High dose rates may not permit repair because of the short time period over which the radiation is given. High-LET radiations do not show a dose-rate effect. This is not surprising, due to the dense ionizations produced by high-LET radiations that "hit" enough targets to kill the cell.

Since the dose-rate effect, then, is largely due to changes in repair, different cells and tissues will exhibit different dose-rate effects depending on their repair capacities. In general, cells and tissues whose survival curves have large shoulders would be expected to show large dose-rate effects, whereas those with small shoulders would be expected to exhibit small dose-rate effects. Such a comparison is shown in Figure 5–5 using lethality at 30 days after total body irradiation or lethality at 9 months after thoracic irradiation only as assays of bone marrow damage and lung damage, respectively. The survival curves for these two tissues differ in that the bone marrow has a long straight initial shoulder while the initial shoulder region for lung is broad and curvy. Reducing the dose rate from 1.8 Gy/min (180 rad/min) to 0.025 Gy/min (2.5 rad/min) has a large effect on lung response, but a minimal effect on bone marrow, as predicted from the shapes of the survival curves for the two tissues.

CHEMICAL FACTORS

Radiation Sensitizers—Oxygen

Many chemicals can change the response of cells to radiation. Some of these chemicals enhance response—these are termed *radiosensitizers*. Chemicals that diminish response are termed *radioprotectors*.

A true radiosensitizer is one that increases the cell-killing effect of a given dose of radiation. Many chemicals have been found that fit this criterion; however, the one that has the most dramatic effect and has been shown to universally enhance radiation response is oxygen. The

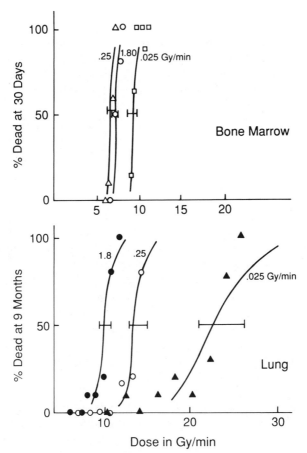

FIG 5–5.
The effect of a range of dose rates from 1.8 to 0.025 Gy/min on bone marrow damage and lung damage as measured by lethality. There is a large dose-rate effect for lung, whereas the dose rate effect is minimal for bone marrow, reflecting the differences in shape of the underlying survival curves of the putative target cell for these two tissues.

universality of this radiosensitizer is attested to by the fact that not only does it enhance the radiation response of mammalian cells in tissue culture, but its effects have been observed in all classes of organisms—from bacteria to whole organisms. Because of its universal and dramatic effect, the response of cells to radiation in the presence of oxygen has been given a specific name—*oxygen effect.*

An interesting facet of the oxygen effect was observed from experiments in which the timing of the delivery of oxygen varied, i.e., oxygen was given either pre-irradiation, postirradiation, or simultaneously with radiation. In these situations, oxygen was found to be most effective when administered simultaneously with radiation; oxygen administered either before or after irradiation did not produce as dramatic a response. These observations led investigators to postulate the mechanism of the oxygen effect. Because the interaction of radiation with matter is a rapid process, and because oxygen was found to be most effective when administered simultaneously with radiation, the effects of oxygen were postulated to involve the reaction of radiation at the chemical level. Although the mechanism of oxygen enhancement of radiation response has been studied extensively, it is still not totally understood. Several theories have been advanced, two of which are most widely accepted:

1. The first hypothesis involves the free radicals formed as a result of radiation interaction with the water content of a cell. Believed to be responsible for a large portion of radiation damage, oxygen may either enhance the formation of free radicals or draw the existing free radicals into chain reactions, producing new, highly damaging radical species.
2. Another mechanism postulated for the sensitizing properties of oxygen is that many of the chemical changes that occur as a result of irradiation are reversible if oxygen is not present. However, if oxygen is present, it may block these restoration processes, thus increasing damage in the cell.

It is generally accepted that oxygen acts at the level of the free radicals that are formed as a result of radiation interaction with the water in the cell. If oxygen were not present, many of these ionized target molecules could repair themselves. Oxygen "fixes" the damage, in that it makes the damage permanent.

Figure 5–6 shows radiation survival curves for the same population of cells, one in the presence of oxygen (aerated) and one in the absence of oxygen (hypoxic). The curve of cells irradiated in oxygen exhibits two changes:

1. The shoulder region of the curve is smaller.
2. The slope of the exponential portion of the curve is steeper, resulting in a decreased D_o dose.

Because oxygen increases the amount of damage through increased free radical formation or by blocking restoration processes, more targets are lethally affected per given dose of radiation. This results in an enhanced response reflected by these changes in the survival curve, indicating an increase in radiosensitivity in oxygenated conditions.

The enhancement of the response of cells to radiation in the presence of oxygen does not increase in an unlimited fashion, however (Fig 5–7). Oxygen concentration is measured by the pressure it exerts and is termed *oxygen tension*; the units of measurement are millimeters of mercury. The response occurs with oxygen tensions between 0 and 20

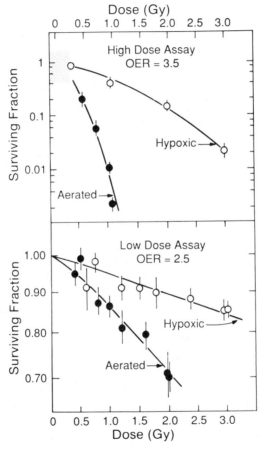

FIG 5–6.
Diagrammatic representation of the effect of oxygen on surviving fraction of cells irradiated over a high dose range or over a low dose range. Based on these data, it is suggested that the OER is not constant over the whole dose range but becomes smaller as the dose is decreased. (From Palcic B, Skarsgard LD: Reduced oxygen enhancement ratio at low doses of ionizing radiation. *Radiat Res* 1984, 100:328–339; and Hall EJ: *Radiobiology for the Radiologist,* ed 3. Philadelphia, JB Lippincott, 1988. Used by permission.)

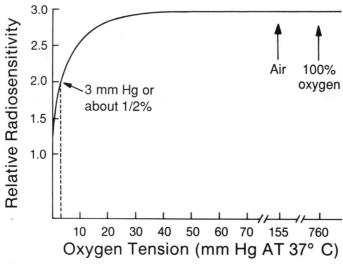

FIG 5–7.
Dependence of radiosensitivity on oxygen concentration illustrating the limitations of the oxygen effect with increasing oxygen tension. The sensitivity is maximum at ~30 mm mercury oxygen tension and does not change very much by increasing the oxygen tension. (From Hall EJ: *Radiobiology for the Radiologist,* ed 3. Philadelphia, JB Lippincott, 1988. Used by permission.)

mm Hg; those greater than 20 to 40 mm Hg (the oxygen tension in air at sea level) result in little further increase in radiation sensitivity.

The term that compares the response of cells or organisms to radiation in the presence and in the absence of oxygen is the *oxygen enhancement ratio (OER)*. OER is defined as the dose of radiation that produces a given biologic response in the absence of oxygen divided by the dose of radiation that produces the same biologic response in the presence of oxygen. For example, if 3 Gy is the D_o of a population of cells exposed under hypoxic conditions (decreased oxygen tension) and 1 Gy is the D_o of the population when oxygen tension is increased, the OER is 3/1, or 3. For mammalian cells, the OER is between 2 and 3, and is generally given as approximately 2.5 after high single doses. Figure 5–6 also compares the OER after high and low doses of x-rays, indicating that OER is not constant over the whole dose range but is lower after low doses. Although hotly debated for a few years, it is now generally accepted that the oxygen enhancement ratio is less after low doses than it is after high doses, as is schematically shown in Figure 5–6.

The oxygen effect is most pronounced with x- and γ-rays (low-LET radiations) and is not as effective with neutrons and alpha particles (high-LET radiations) (Fig 5–8).

Readily explainable by the physical differences between the two types of radiations, the amount of damage produced by high-LET radiations would not be reparable, because it is densely ionizing; therefore, the presence of oxygen would not enhance the radiation response to the same extent as low-LET radiations, which are sparsely ionizing. The OER for high-LET radiations varies between 1.7 and 1.2.

The role of oxygen in the treatment of tumors with radiation has become very important over the past 15 years. This will be discussed further in Chapter 10.

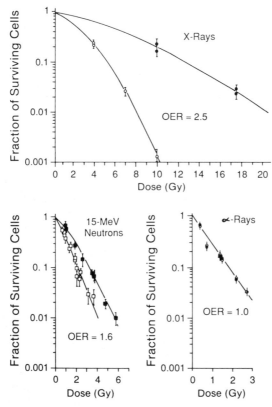

FIG 5–8.
Comparison of the oxygen effect after x-ray, neutron, or α-particle irradiation. Note that the OER is highest after sparsely ionizing radiations (OER = 2.5) than after densely ionizing radiations such as alpha-particles (OER = 1.0). (From Broerse JJ, Barendsen GW, van Kersen GR: Survival of cultured human cells after irradiation with fast neutrons at different energies in hypoxic and oxygenated conditions. *Int J Radiat Biol* 1967; 13:559–572. Used by permission.)

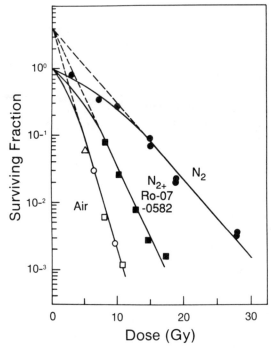

FIG 5–9.
The effect of the radiosensitizer misonidazole (RO-07-0582) on survival as a function of x-ray dose. Note that the addition of misonidazole shifts the hypoxic survival curve close to that of well-aerated cells. (From Adams GE, Flockhart IR, Smithen CE, et al: Electron-affinic sensitization. VII. A correlation between structures, one-electron reduction potentials, and efficiencies of nitroimidazoles as hypoxic cell radiosensitizers. *Radiat Res* 1976; 67:9–20. Used by permission.)

Other Sensitizers

Because of the well-known oxygen effect and its implications in clinical radiotherapy (see Chapter 10), an attempt has been made to find chemicals that mimic oxygen and its effect. The most widely tested of these compounds fall in a class of substances known as the nitrofurans. The most well known of this group of compounds is misonidazole, or RO-07-0582. The effect of misonidazole on aerated and hypoxic Chinese hamster ovary cells is shown in Figure 5–9. When hypoxic cells are irradiated with x-rays in the presence of misonidazole the radiation sensitivity of these cells approaches that of irradiated aerated cells. The compound has no effect on the sensitivity of well-aerated cells. For these reasons, these compounds became of great interest in clinical radiotherapy, as discussed in Chapter 10.

Halogenated pyrimidines are chemical compounds that substitute for the base thymidine in the DNA molecule. Two halogenated pyrimidines that are effective radiosensitizers are 5-bromodeoxyuridine (5-BUDR) and 5-iododeoxyuridine (5-IUDR). When present in a cell, these compounds will be selectively incorporated into DNA in place of thymidine, changing the molecule and thereby rendering it more susceptible to radiation damage. Because the radiation-enhancing effects of these compounds are dependent on their incorporation into DNA, unlike oxygen, they must be present for several cell cycles before irradiation to be effective.

Both these compounds sensitize cells by a factor of 2; in other words, if BUDR is incorporated into DNA, it will take one half the dose to produce the same response as is produced in cells without BUDR. The presence of BUDR has been shown to enhance two cellular responses to radiation: reproductive failure and division delay.

Radiation Protectors

Approximately 20 years ago it was discovered that certain compounds, when present at the time of radiation, had a protective effect on the organism. It was also observed that these compounds had to be present at the time of irradiation to exert the protective effect—if administered immediately following irradiation, no protective effect was noted. These compounds, called radioprotectors, act by reducing the effective dose of radiation to the cells.

One group of compounds with radioprotectant properties consists of chemicals that contain a sulfhydryl group (sulfur and hydrogen bound together, designated SH). Two amino acids in the body belonging to this group of sulfhydryl compounds are cysteine and cysteamine. In fact, cysteine was one of the first compounds found to have radioprotectant properties. The sulfhydryl compound most widely studied is WR-2721. When one of these compounds is given prior to radiation, a larger dose of radiation is necessary to produce the same response as when the compound is not present. This difference in dose for a given response in relation to the presence of the protective compound is called *dose reduction factor (DRF)* or *protection factor (PF)*.

The DRF is defined as the ratio of the radiation dose necessary to produce a given effect in the presence of a protecting compound to the radiation dose necessary to produce the same effect in the absence of the same compound. The DRF for the sulfhydryl-containing compounds is approximately 1.5 to 2.0. If such a compound is present during radiation, almost twice the dose is required to produce the same response as that produced by one half the dose in the absence of the compound (Fig 5–10).

Many hypotheses have been advanced concerning the mechanism of action of these dose-modifying agents. The most generally accepted hypothesis today is that these agents protect either by competing for the radiation-produced free radicals or by giving up a hydrogen atom to ionized molecules in the cell, neutralizing the effects of radiation and restoring the molecule to its original pre-irradiated state.

The sulfhydryl compounds are most efficient with x- and γ-rays and have a negligible effect with high-LET radiations such as alpha particles and neutrons. Thus, the protection observed with these compounds parallels the oxygen effect; these compounds exhibit maximum protection with low-LET radiation and minimum protection with high-LET radiations, just as oxygen exhibits maximum sensitivity with low-LET and minimum sensitivity with high-LET radiations.

The modifying agents discussed above are not in widespread use due to a number of factors. It would seem feasible that radioprotector compounds would be useful in radiation safety for protection against overexposure. However, the concentration of these compounds necessary to protect an organism is toxic, therefore prohibiting their use. In addition, these agents must be present in the cell at the time of

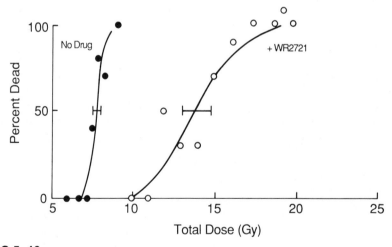

FIG 5–10.
Effect of the administration of the radioprotector WR-2721 on lethality at 30 days after single doses of radiation. The dose for isoeffect, in this case $LD_{50/30}$, in the absence of the compound is 7.8 Gy, whereas the $LD_{50/30}$ is 13.8 Gy if the thiol-compound is present before irradiation. Thus the protection factor (or dose reduction factor) is about 2.

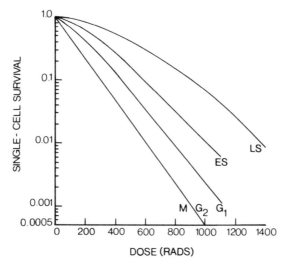

FIG 5–11.
Graph illustrating the effect of cell cycle position on cell survival of a synchronous population of cells. M and G_2 periods are the most radiosensitive, whereas early S period (ES) and late S period (LS) are the most resistant. (From Sinclair WK: Cyclic responses in mammalian cells in vitro. *Radiat Res* 1968; 33:620. Used by permission.)

irradiation, not after irradiation, making them useless for treatment in cases of accidental overexposure.

Another potential application of radioprotectors is to protect normal tissues in the treatment field when radiation is used in the treatment of cancer. This topic is discussed in Chapter 10.

BIOLOGIC FACTORS

Cell Cycle

In addition to chemical and physical factors that alter the cellular radiation response, there are some important biologic factors that also modify the response. One biologic factor that has a great influence on cellular response is the position of the cell in the cell cycle at the time of irradiation. By using techniques that synchronize a population of cells (place all cells in one phase of the cell cycle), it is possible to observe the responses of cells in various phases.

A summary of the experimental findings indicates that cells are more radiosensitive when irradiated in G_2 and M periods, less sensitive in G_1 period and least sensitive (most radioresistant) during DNA synthesis (Fig 5–11). In general, M is considered to be the most radiosensitive phase in the cell cycle and S the most resistant.

Division delay, a dose-dependent cellular response, is directly related to the position of the cell in the cell cycle. Low doses of radiation affect cells in the most radiosensitive phases of the cell cycle (G_2 and M), delaying their progression through mitosis for a given period of time. Higher doses, affecting cells in all phases of the cycle, both radiosensitive and radioresistant, produce a longer mitotic delay.

Intracellular Repair

A second biologic factor that influences cellular response is the capability of cells to repair sublethal damage, i.e., recover from radiation injury (as discussed in Chapter 3). Elkind and Sutton-Gilbert determined that when the same total dose is administered in fractions separated by a period of time, the number of cells surviving increased with the time between fractions. In addition, the survival curve after the second dose exhibited the same D_o, n, and D_q as the survival curve following the first dose of radiation (Fig 5–12).

In essence, cells surviving the first dose fraction respond as unirradiated cells to the second fraction. This observation was interpreted as meaning that radiation damage had been repaired between the first

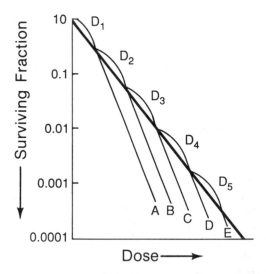

FIG 5–12.
The effect of dose fractionation on cell survival. After each succeeding dose fraction (D_1, D_2, D_3, etc.) the curve exhibits the same shoulder, slope, and extrapolation number, indicating that within a given period of time damage is repaired. (From Elkind MM, Whitmore GF: *Radiobiology of Cultured Mammalian Cells.* New York, Gordon & Breach, 1967. Used by permission.)

and second doses, indicating that cells have the capability of recovering from sublethal injury (injury not resulting in death). For this reason a higher total dose is necessary to produce the same biologic response when the dose is fractionated than when given acutely. In addition, this process appears to be completed in the cell within 24 hours postirradiation.

The ability of the cell to repair intracellular radiation damage has implications for radiation therapy and will be discussed further in Chapter 10.

REFERENCES

1. Adams GE, Flockhart IR, Smithen CE, et al: Electron-affinic sensitization. VII. A correlation between structures, one-electron reduction potentials, and efficiencies of nitroimidazoles as hypoxic cell radiosensitizers. *Radiat Res* 1976; 67:9–20.
2. Arena V: *Ionizing Radiations and Life.* St Louis, CV Mosby, 1971.
3. Bacq ZM, Alexander P: *Fundamentals of Radiobiology,* ed 2. New York, Pergamon Press, 1961.
4. Barendsen GW: Impairment of the proliferative capacity of human cells in culture by alpha particles with differing linear energy transfer. *Int J Radiat Biol,* 1964, 8:453.
5. Barendsen GW, et al: Effects of different ionizing radiations on human cells in tissue culture. II. Biological experiments. *Radiat Res* 1960; 13:841.
6. Bedford JS, Hall EJ: Survival of HeLa cells cultured in vitro and exposed to protracted gamma irradiation. *Int J Radiat Biol* 1963; 7:377.
7. Bedford JS, Mitchell JB: Dose-rate effects in synchronous mammalian cells in culture. *Radiat Res* 1973; 54:316–327.
8. Belli JA, et al: Radiation recovery response in mammalian tumor cells in vivo. *Nature* 1966; 211:662.
9. Belli JA, et al: Radiation response of mammalian tumor cells. I. Repair of sublethal damage in vivo. *J Natl Cancer Inst* 1967; 38:673.
10. Berry RJ: Modification of radiation effects. *Radiol Clin North Am* 1965; 3:249.
11. Berry RJ, Cohen AB: Some observations on the reproductive capacity of mammalian tumor cells exposed in vivo to gamma radiation at low dose rates. *Br J Radiol* 1962; 35:489.
12. Berry RJ, et al: Reproductive capacity of mammalian tumor cells irradiated in vivo with cyclotron produced fast neutrons. *Br J Radiol* 1965, 38:613.
13. Broerse JJ, Barendsen GW: Current topics. *Radiat Res Q* 1973; 8:305–350.

14. Broerse JJ, Barendsen GW, van Kersen GR: Survival of cultured human cells after irradiation with fast neutrons at different energies in hypoxic and oxygenated conditions. *Int J Radiat Biol* 1967; 13:559–572.

15. Brown JM, et al: Preferential radiosensitization of mouse sarcoma relative to normal skin by chronic intra-arterial infusion of halogenated pyrimidine analogs. *J Natl Cancer Inst* 1971; 47:75.

16. Canti RG, Spear FG: The effect of gamma irradiation on cell division in tissue culture in vitro, Part II. *Proc R Soc Lond [Biol]* 1929; 105:93.

17. Elkind MM, Sutton-Gilbert H: Radiation response of mammalian cells grown in culture. I. Repair of x-ray damage in surviving Chinese hamster cells. *Radiat Res* 1960; 13:556.

18. Elkind MM, et al: Actinomycin D; suppression of recovery in x-irradiated mammalian cells. *Science* 1964; 143:1454.

19. Elkind MM, et al: Radiation response in mammalian cells in culture. V. Temperature dependence of the repair of x-ray damage in surviving cells (aerobic and hypoxic). *Radiat Res* 1965; 25:359.

20. Field SB: The relative biological effectiveness of fast neutrons for mammalian tissues. *Radiology* 1969; 93:915.

21. Hall EJ: Radiation dose rate: A factor of importance in radiobiology and radiotherapy. *Br J Radiol* 1972; 45:81.

22. Hall EJ: *Radiobiology for the Radiologist*, ed 3. Philadelphia, JB Lippincott, 1988.

23. Hall EJ, Bedford JS: Dose-rate: Its effect on the survival of HeLa cells irradiated with gamma rays. *Radiat Res* 1964; 22:305.

24. Hornsey S: *Advances in Radiobiology.* New York, Academic Press, 1957.

25. Howard-Flanders P, Alper T: The sensitivity of micro-organisms to radiation under controlled gas conditions. *Radiat Res* 1957; 7:518.

26. Lea DE: *Actions of Radiations on Living Cells*, ed 2. Cambridge, Cambridge University Press, 1962.

27. Littbrand B, Revesz L: Effects of a second exposure to x-rays on post-irradiation recovery. *Nature* 1967; 214:841.

28. Mohler WC, Elkind MM: Radiation response in mammalian cells grown in culture. III. Modification of x-ray survival of Chinese hamster cells by 5-bromo-deoxyuridine. *Exp Cell Res* 1963; 30:481.

29. Nakken KF: Radical scavengers in radioprotection, in Ebert M, Howard A (eds): *Current Topics in Radiation Research.* Amsterdam, North Holland Publishing Co, 1965.

30. Palcic B, Skarsgard LD: Reduced oxygen enhancement ratio at low doses of ionizing radiation. *Radiat Res* 1984; 100:328–339.

31. Read J: The effect of ionizing radiation on the broad bean root. XI. The dependence of alpha ray sensitivity on dissolved oxygen. *Br J Radiol* 1952; 25:651.

32. Read J: Mode of action of x-ray doses given with different oxygen concentrations. *Br J Radiol* 1952; 25:335.

33. Sinclair WK: Cyclic responses in mammalian cells in vitro. *Radiat Res* 1968; 33:620.

34. Sinclair WK: Dependence of radiosensitivity upon cell age, in *Time and Dose Relationships in Radiation Biology as Applied to Radiotherapy,* Proceedings of the Conference, Carmel, California, September 1969. BNL Report 50203-C-57, Biology in Medicine TID 4500; Upton, NY, Brookhaven National Laboratory, 1969.

35. Sinclair WK: Radiation survival in synchronous and asynchronous Chinese hamster cells in vitro, in *Biological Aspects of Radiation Quality,* Proceedings of the Second IAEA Panel, Vienna, 1967. Vienna, IAEA, 1968.

36. Sinclair WK, Morton RA: X-ray sensitivity during the cell generation cycle of cultured Chinese hamster cells. *Radiat Res* 1966; 29:450.

37. Terasima R, Tolmach LJ: X-ray sensitivity and DNA synthesis in synchronous populations of HeLa cells. *Science* 1963; 140:490.

38. Wright EA, Howard-Flanders P: The influence of oxygen on the radiosensitivity of mammalian tissues. *Acta Radiol (Stockholm)* 1957; 48:26.

Chapter 6 ——————————

Radiation Pathology

Cardiovascular System
  Vasculature
  Heart
    Diagnostic Radiology and Nuclear Medicine
    Radiation Therapy
  Growing Bone and Cartilage
    Diagnostic Radiology and Nuclear Medicine
    Radiation Therapy
  Liver
    Diagnostic Radiology and Nuclear Medicine
    Radiation Therapy
  Respiratory System
    Diagnostic Radiology and Nuclear Medicine
    Radiation Therapy
  Urinary System
    Diagnostic Radiology and Nuclear Medicine
    Radiation Therapy
  Central Nervous System
    Diagnostic Radiology and Nuclear Medicine
    Radiation Therapy

As discussed in Chapter 5, normal tissues can be divided into two categories, acutely responding and late responding, based solely on the time in which they express damage after irradiation. However, this classification does not describe what is observed, i.e., the morphologic and structural changes that occur after irradiation. The pathologic changes that occur after irradiation of specific organs are the topic of this chapter. The response of the total body to an acute dose of radiation will be discussed in the next chapter.

The underlying assumption throughout this chapter (as in all previous chapters) is that cell death, whether via reproductive failure or interphase death, and subsequent loss of cells from the organ is the initial event that leads to the visible changes. In most cases the visible effects of radiation on the morphology of an organ are not unique—without the knowledge that radiation exposure has occurred, the observed changes would not implicate radiation as the causative agent. Many other types of trauma will produce the same changes.

"ACUTE" vs. CHRONIC EFFECTS

The morphologic response of an organ or tissue after irradiation occurs in two general phases, often referred to as "acute" and "late" effects. In this chapter the term chronic effect will be used rather than "late" effect to avoid confusion with the true "late" effects of radiation to be discussed in Chapter 8. These terms, which refer to what is observed, are not to be confused with the terms "acutely" responding and "late" responding normal tissues (see Chapter 4), which refer only to *when* the damage is expressed, not to *what* this damage looks like.

The first phase, i.e., the "acute" effect, may occur soon after irradiation as in "acutely" responding normal tissues, or at long times after irradiation as in "late" responding normal tissues, dependent on the turnover kinetics of the putative target cells in the parenchyma of the tissue. However, regardless of the time after irradiation that this initial response occurs, the cause is the same: depletion of *parenchymal* cells specific to the tissue. Examples of an acute response in two tissues which is expressed at vastly different times are the initial response in the esophagus, esophagitis, and in the lung, pneumonitis, acutely responding and late responding normal tissues, respectively. Esophagitis appears within the first month after irradiation, whereas pneumonitis is not manifested until 3 months or longer after irradiation. However, damage in both tissues is due to depletion of parenchymal cells, basal cells in the mucosa of the esophagus, and (most likely), type 2 pneumocytes of the alveolar epithelium of the lung. These changes may be reversible or irreversible, depending on dose and the proliferative potential of the target cells.

Chronic (late) effects may occur either (1) as a consequence of irreversible and subsequently progressive early changes, or (2) due to depletion of critical *nonparenchymal* cells, perhaps in the stroma or the vasculature. Chronic effects occurring as a consequence of severe acute effects (as in item 1 above) can be termed "secondary" chronic effects, and those that are a result of depletion of nonparenchymal cells (as in item 2 above) can be termed "primary" chronic effects. The former are dependent on the acute effects, whereas the latter would be independent of the acute effects. Both types are permanent, irreversible, and most likely progressive. Because secondary chronic effects are a consequence of severe acute effects, it is likely that they appear sooner and progress more quickly than primary chronic effects. The latter would appear at a time consistent with the very slow turnover of the critical target cell population. These changes would appear at long times after the acute response had subsided and would progress over a longer period of time, perhaps, even, for years. Chronic effects can occur years after radiotherapy is completed. In general, whether a primary or secondary chronic effect occurs is a function of the type of healing that occurs in the organ.

HEALING

Healing of a tissue or organ occurs by one of two means: *regeneration*, the replacement of damaged cells in the organ by the same cell type present before radiation; or *repair*, the replacement of the depleted original cells by a different cell type. Regeneration results in a total or partial reversal of early radiation changes, actually restoring the organ to its pre-irradiated state both morphologically and functionally. In this situation, any chronic changes would be of a primary nature, i.e., due to depletion of a different cell type in a different part of the tissue.

On the other hand, catastrophic and irreversible acute changes heal by *repair*. This process does not restore the organ to its pre-irradiated condition, thus producing a secondary chronic response. Repair of radiation damage usually does not contribute to the ability of the organ to perform its function.

Healing of either type is not an absolutely certain event, and under conditions that produce massive and extensive damage, may not occur, resulting in tissue necrosis.

The type of healing that occurs in an organ following radiation is a function of both dose and specific organ irradiated. Although repair can occur in any organ, whether acutely or late responding, regeneration occurs after low, moderate, and even high doses in organs whose cells are either actively dividing or retain the capability of division, such as skin, small intestine, and bone marrow (acutely responding normal tissues). In these organs, repair occurs *only* after high doses that destroy large numbers of parenchymal cells, rendering regeneration impossible or incomplete. On the other hand, late responding organs consisting of slowly dividing cells (e.g., lung and kidney) have minimal regenerative capabilities; therefore, moderate and high doses of radiation result mostly in repair.

An important factor in understanding the responses of different organs to radiation is time. Acutely responding normal tissues will show changes sooner than late responding organs exposed to the same dose; in fact, an acutely responding organ may manifest a severe response, while a minimal response may be observed in a late responding organ exposed to the same dose and observed at the same time postexposure. However, at a later time the reverse situation may be true. For example, irradiation of one lung (late responding) and the overlying skin (acutely responding) with a single dose of 20 Gy produces marked changes in the skin at 6 months postexposure, but lung changes are less severe. Observations at 1 year postexposure reveal minimal skin changes, but now the irradiated lung exhibits severe changes.

CLINICAL FACTORS INFLUENCING RESPONSE

Because the response of each organ will be related to the three medical specialties using radiation, a word is necessary at this point concerning the doses received from each of these specialties. Low doses (less than 1 Gy) are generally delivered to only a portion of the patient's body by diagnostic radiography, fluoroscopy, and nuclear medicine. Patient doses in radiation therapy are much higher, usually on the order of 40 to 60 Gy. However, the total dose in radiotherapy is fractionated; it is split into many small daily doses administered over a period of time (generally 2 Gy/day over 4 to 6 weeks, a "standard" fractionation schedule). Although the basis of dose fractionation in radiotherapy will be thoroughly discussed in Chapter 10, it is sufficient for our purposes here to realize that a dose administered in multiple fractions is biologically less effective than a single dose of the same magnitude (Chapters 3 and 4). In other words, most organs show less response if the total dose is fractionated than if given as a single dose. This is an extremely important point to keep in mind throughout this chapter to avoid misunderstandings about organ response in radiotherapy.

Another vital factor in understanding clinical organ response is the relationship of volume. In general, although irradiation of part of an organ will elicit the same morphologic response in that specific area as in the whole organ exposed to the same dose, these two situations will have different consequences to the life of the individual. Irradiation of the whole organ may be life-threatening; however, a sufficient amount of undamaged organ may remain after only partial irradiation of a critical organ to ensure function and, therefore, life of the individual. Since this factor is of obvious clinical concern, particularly in radiotherapy, volume effects will be briefly discussed when appropriate.

GENERAL ORGAN CHANGES

In general, acute changes in most organs are characterized by inflammation, edema, and hemorrhage and a denudation of mucosal surfaces. Chronic changes consist of fibrosis, atrophy (decrease in size of an organ), ulceration, stricture, stenosis, and obstruction. Pathologically, it is not possible to distinguish between secondary and primary chronic changes, and time is most likely the critical factor in distinguishing between these two chronic effects. Necrosis is the result of failure to repair damage by any means and represents the ultimate secondary chronic effect.

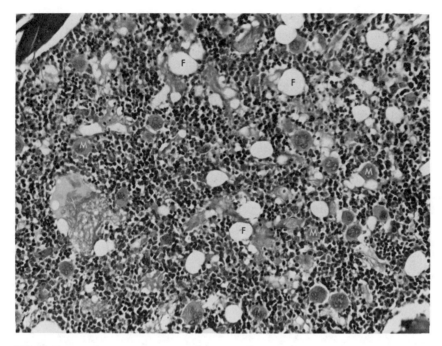

FIG 6–1.
Photomicrograph of normal bone marrow from rat sternum showing both fat cells *(F)* and megakaryocytes *(M)*; a special stain, Giemsa, would be necessary to identify the remaining red and white cells present. (H & E stain, magnification × 250.)

Specific organ response will be discussed by system. Because the general response of a system is determined by the most radiosensitive organ in that system, attention will be focused on the organ or organs that account for the changes.

HEMOPOIETIC SYSTEM

The hemopoietic system includes the bone marrow, circulating blood, lymph nodes, spleen, and thymus (these last three organs are termed *lymphoid* organs).

Bone Marrow

Bone marrow tissues include the parenchymal cells of the marrow, consisting of precursor (stem) cells and material end cells in the circulating blood, fat cells, and a connective tissue stroma. There are two types of marrow in the adult: red and yellow. Red marrow contains a large number of stem cells, in addition to fat cells (Fig 6–1), and is primarily responsible for supplying mature, functional cells to the circulating blood. In adults, red marrow is present in the following sites: ribs, ends of long bones, vertebrae, sternum, and skull bones. Yellow marrow, consisting primarily of fat cells with very few stem cells, is not active in supplying mature cells to the circulating blood and, due to the fat content, is commonly termed "fatty" marrow. Fetal bone marrow is predominantly red marrow, whereas in the adult, red marrow is located in specific sites.

The primary effect of radiation on the bone marrow is to decrease the number of stem cells. Low doses result in a slight decrease with recovery (stem cell repopulation of the marrow) occurring within a few weeks postexposure. Moderate and high doses produce a more severe depletion of cells in the bone marrow, resulting in either a longer period of recovery (time before repopulation of the marrow is complete) and/or less recovery—manifested as a permanent decrease in stem cell numbers and an increase in the amount of fat and connective tissue (Fig 6–2).

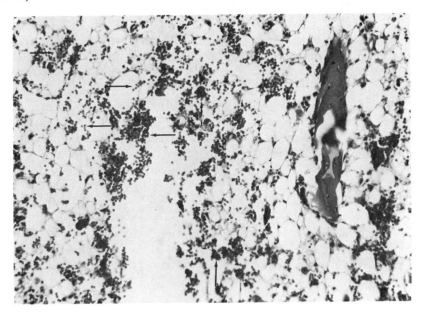

FIG 6–2.
Photomicrograph of bone marrow from rat sternum exposed to total body dose of 10 Gy, 5 days postirradiation, exhibiting overall hypocellularity and relative increase in fat cells. Note the absence of megakaryocytes, clumps of hyperchromatic, pyknotic cells *(arrows),* and red blood cells *(arrows),* a result of hemorrhage. (H & E stain, magnification × 250.)

Although all stem cells in the bone marrow are very radiosensitive, variations in sensitivity exist among these different cells. Erythroblasts (precursor cells for red blood cells) are the most radiosensitive; myelocytes (precursors for some white blood cells) are second in sensitivity; and megakaryocytes (precursors for platelets) are the least radiosensitive. This variation in sensitivity is manifested as a difference in the time of depression of counts in the different stem cells as follows: erythroblasts decrease first and return to normal approximately 1 week after a moderate dose, myelocytes are depressed in the same time period as erythroblasts but require a longer time to recover (2 to 6 weeks), and depression of megakaryocytes occurs at 1 to 2 weeks postexposure requiring a recovery time of 2 to 6 weeks. Low doses result in decreased stem cell numbers and fast recovery, whereas a more severe decrease in numbers in all cell lines occurs after moderate and high doses, with either slow recovery or incomplete recovery of cell numbers relative to pre-irradiated values.

Circulating Blood

With the exception of lymphocytes, the cells in the circulating blood are resistant to radiation (they are nondividing, differentiated cells). However, the circulating blood reflects radiation damage in the bone marrow; as the number of stem cells in the marrow decreases, a corresponding decrease will be exhibited in the number of the respective, mature circulating cells.

The reflection of bone marrow damage in circulating blood cells is dependent on two factors:

1. The sensitivity of the different stem cells.
2. The lifespan of each cell type in the circulating blood.

Although both these factors are important, the latter is more significant in terms of the time of appearance of changes in the circulating blood. All cells in the circulating blood have a finite lifespan (i.e., at certain times they die and must be replaced), varying on the average from 24 hours (granulocytes) to 120 days (erythrocytes). Damage to the respective stem cells in the bone marrow will be reflected in the circulating blood only when the mature cells die and must be replaced.

Lymphocytes decrease first (counts are affected by doses as low as 0.1 Gy), neutrophils are second (doses of 0.5 Gy are necessary to produce a decrease), and platelets and RBCs are third (at doses greater than 0.5 Gy; Fig 6–3). Lymphocyte counts will approach zero within a few days

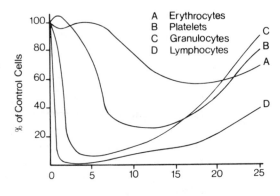

A Erythrocytes
B Platelets
C Granulocytes
D Lymphocytes

Time in Days after Radiation

FIG 6–3.
Illustration of decrease in number of various blood cells in circulating blood of rat exposed
to a moderate dose of total body irradiation. Note the order and time of depletion and recovery
of the four cell lines. (From Casarett AP: *Radiation Biology.* Englewood Cliffs, New Jersey,
Prentice-Hall, 1968. Used by permission.)

following a moderate dose, with full recovery occurring within a few
months postexposure. Lower doses produce a slight depression of lymphocytes, followed by recovery and a return of the lymphocyte count
to pre-irradiated values.

Granulocytes counts fall to minimal values approximately 1 week
following a moderate dose. However, recovery begins soon and neu-
trophil counts approach normal values within a month postexposure.

The lower doses in the moderate range will have a minimal effect
on platelets and RBCs, but the higher doses of this range result in
marked depression of these cells. Recovery begins later in these cell
lines, approximately the 4th week postexposure, and is usually complete within a few months.

A decrease in the numbers of these various cells has implications
for life. Granulocytes and lymphocytes are part of the body's defense
mechanism and are important in fighting infection; a decreased number
of these cells increases the individual's susceptibility to infection. A
decrease in platelets (necessary for blood clotting) results in hemorrhage. Anemia follows depression of RBCs and is compounded by hemorrhage throughout the body.

Diagnostic Radiology.—Radiation doses in the diagnostic range
pose no *major* hazard to the blood and blood-forming organs of the
patient or occupationally exposed personnel, in terms of decreased cell
counts. However, chromosome changes have been observed in circulating lymphocytes following doses in this range.

Nuclear Medicine.—Because radionuclides are primarily given intravenously for diagnostic purposes, the circulating blood is exposed to radiation. Chromosomal changes may occur as a result of these doses, but the probabilities are small because of the small amount of radionuclide given and the consequent low dose to which the blood is exposed. In addition, any chromosome changes in the circulating cells will not be propagated due to the finite lifespan of the cells involved. Whether changes occur in stem cells is not known.

Radiation Therapy.—When active bone marrow is in the treatment volume, doses in the therapeutic range will cause a depression of all blood cells, particularly white cells. For this reason blood counts should be routinely obtained on all patients receiving radiotherapy, particularly those receiving radiation to large volumes of tissue—e.g., in the treatment of Hodgkin's disease and ovarian cancer—or those in which the treatment field includes a large amount of red marrow.

SKIN

The skin consists of an outer layer (epidermis), a layer of connective tissue (dermis), and a subcutaneous layer of fat and connective tissue. The skin is supplied with nutrients by blood vessels and contains specialized structures, e.g., hair follicles, sebaceous glands, and sweat glands, which arise in the dermis.

The epidermis is made up of layers of cells consisting of both mature, nondividing cells (at the surface) and immature, dividing cells (at the base of the epidermis—the "basal layer"). Cells are periodically lost from the surface of the skin and must be replaced by division of cells in the basal layer. The specific characteristics of the basal cells in the epidermis render the skin sensitive to radiation.

Acute changes in the skin following a moderate or high dose of radiation are inflammation, erythema (redness of the skin), and dry or moist desquamation (denudation of the skin surface). The skin erythema produced by radiation is not unlike that seen after prolonged exposure to the sun. Produced by an acute dose of 10 Gy, this particular reaction was at one time used as a yardstick to measure the amount of radiation to which an individual had been exposed. The term denoting that dose of radiation that causes this skin erythema is the *skin erythema dose (SED)*.

Moderate doses permit healing to occur in the epidermis by regenerative means, resulting in minimal chronic changes. However, chronic changes such as atrophy (thinning of the epidermis, Fig 6–4), fibrosis,

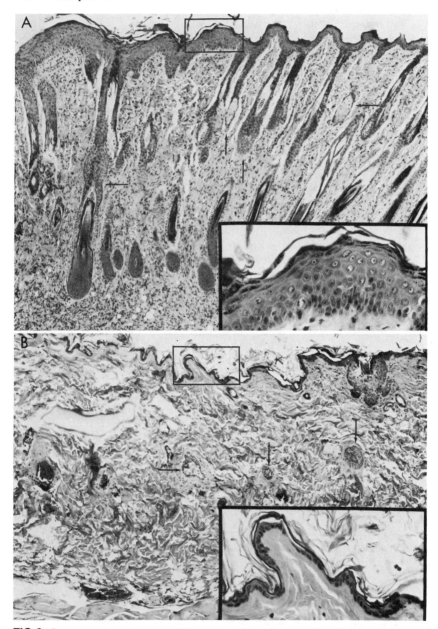

FIG 6–4.
Photomicrograph of normal (**A**) and irradiated (**B**) rat skin exposed to 20 Gy to a localized
area of the body; the animal was sacrificed 1 year postexposure. **Insets** show magnified
views of the epidermis. Note the number of cell layers in the epidermis of the unirradiated
animal, while that of the irradiated animal consists of only one cell layer. Normal skin contains
numerous hair follicles and sebaceous glands *(arrows),* but the irradiated area contains only
fibrotic accessory structures *(arrows).* (H & E stain; magnification × 40; inserts, magnification
× 500.)

decreased or increased pigmentation, ulceration, necrosis, and cancer (the latter late effect appearing many years postexposure) may be seen after exposure to high doses (Fig 6–5).

Accessory Structures

Hair follicles, as an actively growing tissue, are radiosensitive, with moderate doses causing a temporary epilation or alopecia (synonyms for hair loss), while high doses may cause permanent epilation. Sebaceous and sweat glands are relatively radioresistant; damage after high doses produces glandular atrophy and fibrosis, resulting in minimal or no function (Fig 6–4).

Diagnostic Radiology.—Doses from diagnostic radiographic and fluoroscopic procedures today pose no hazard in terms of the above-described changes (providing, of course, that proper precautions are taken). However, many of these changes, particularly erythema and cancer, occurred on the hands of pioneer workers in radiology. There are known cases of erythema produced in patients as a result of failure to place filtration in the beam.

Nuclear Medicine.—No early or late skin changes have been observed on the hands of occupationally exposed persons in nuclear medicine, but hand doses are increasing due to both an increase in the number of procedures performed and the amounts of certain radionuclides used, e.g., ^{99m}Tc.

Radiation Therapy.—Both the early and chronic changes described above have been observed in patients receiving radiation therapy, particularly when orthovoltage units were in widespread use. With today's high-energy units, chronic skin changes are minimal; fractionated doses in the range of 60 Gy in 6 weeks usually produce only atrophy of the irradiated area. Although atrophy does decrease the ability of the irradiated area to withstand trauma of any type, this is a relatively minor effect that can be circumvented if further treatment of the area is necessary. Severe necrosis is extremely rare today, and is never produced deliberately in practice. It may occur in an individual who is particularly sensitive to radiation due to unusual treatment protocols or to failure to follow the prescribed treatment plan (e.g., wedges not placed in the radiation beam when specified).

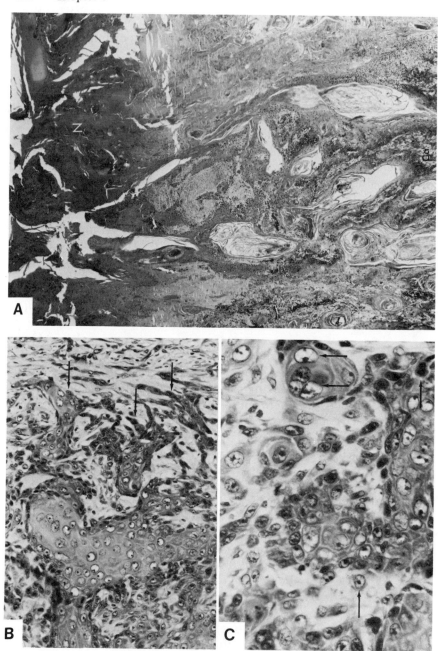

FIG 6–5.
A, ulcerated, necrotic *(N)* rat skin that was exposed to 20 Gy to a localized body area and sacrificed 1 year postexposure. Beneath the ulcerated area is a carcinoma showing **(B)** invasion *(arrows)* and **(C)** cells with atypical nuclei and mitotic figures *(arrows).* (H & E stain; A magnification × 40; B magnification × 150; C magnification × 350.)

DIGESTIVE SYSTEM

The alimentary canal consists, in part, of the mouth, esophagus, stomach, small intestine, large intestine, and rectum. The system is a closed tube throughout the body lined by a mucous membrane, which, like the skin, contains layers of cells, some of which are dividing and undifferentiated (radiosensitive), and some of which are nondividing and differentiated (radioresistant).

Moderate to high doses of radiation produce inflammation in the mucous membranes of the oral cavity (mucositis) and esophagus (esophagitis); however, healing occurs with minimal chronic changes after moderate doses, while high doses result in atrophy, ulceration, fibrosis, and esophageal stricture.

The stomach appears to be more sensitive than the esophagus, with moderately high doses producing ulceration, atrophy, and fibrosis. The small intestine is the most radiosensitive portion of the gastrointestinal (GI) tract. The lining of the small intestine forms fingerlike projections (villi) which aid in the absorption of digested materials into the bloodstream. The cells of this lining are nondividing and are sloughed (lost) from the tips of the villi daily and replaced by cells that arise from the crypts of Lieberkühn (nests of cells at the base of the villi—a rapidly dividing, undifferentiated stem cell population). Radiation damage in the small intestine is a result of damage to these cells.

Moderate doses of radiation result in shortening of the villi due to a killing of the crypt cells, followed by regeneration of these cells with a corresponding repopulation and healing of the villi. After high doses, more cells are killed, minimal recovery occurs, the villi become shortened and flattened and the intestine may become denuded (complete loss of cells) leading to ulceration, hemorrhage, fibrosis, and necrosis (Fig 6–6).

Changes in and damage to the large intestine and rectum after high doses are similar to those already outlined; the rectum, along with the esophagus, appears to be much more resistant to radiation than the stomach or small intestine. Chronic effects in the intestine consist of intestinal strictures, obstruction, and adhesions.

Diagnostic Radiology and Nuclear Medicine.—Neither diagnostic radiography and fluoroscopy nor radionuclide procedures deliver doses of a magnitude great enough to result in the type of changes detailed above.

Radiation Therapy.—Changes in the digestive system have implications for radiotherapy. Esophagitis and mucositis commonly occur during and after treatment at doses of 10 to 20 Gy, but minimal chronic effects are observed even at total doses of 60 to 70 Gy. Irradiation of the small intestine is often unavoidable when treating certain diseases (e.g., ovarian cancer by moving-strip or whole-abdomen technique), but chronic effects are minimal. Early effects are often manifested by symptoms such as nausea, vomiting, and diarrhea. The incidence and severity of chronic effects in different parts of the GI tract increase with the total fractionated dose reflecting, the sensitivity of the individual

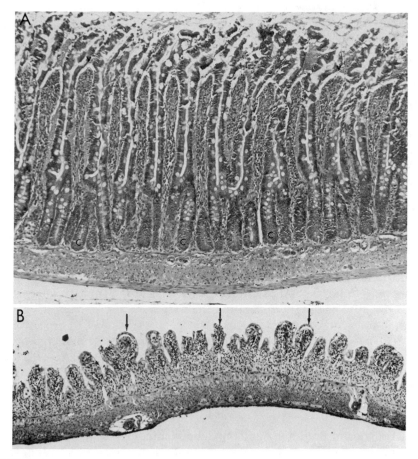

FIG 6–6.
Small intestine of a rat exposed to 20 Gy total body dose, sacrificed 5 days postirradiation. **A,** normal intestinal mucosa with typical long villi *(V),* and numerous crypts *(C).* **B,** edema and blunting of the villi, loss of crypts, and almost total denudation of the intestinal mucosa *(arrows).* (H & E stain, magnification × 40.)

organs. For example, 9% of the patients receiving 50 Gy to the colon develop partial obstruction, while at doses greater than 60 Gy, 25% develop this chronic change.

REPRODUCTIVE SYSTEM

Male

Most of the tissues of the male reproductive system, with the exception of the testes, are radioresistant. The testes contain both non-dividing, differentiated, radioresistant cells (mature spermatozoa) and rapidly dividing, undifferentiated, radiosensitive cells (immature spermatogonia). It is this latter cell population in the testes that accounts for the radiosensitivity of the system.

The primary effect of radiation on the male reproductive system is damage and depopulation of the spermatogonia, eventually resulting in depletion of mature sperm in the testes, a process termed *maturation depletion* (Fig 6–7). A variable period of fertility occurs after testicular irradiation, attributable to the radioresistance of the mature sperm, and is followed by temporary or permanent sterility, depending on the dose. Sterility is due to a loss of the immature spermatogonia, which divide and replace the mature sperm lost from the testes. Permanent sterility can be produced by an acute radiation dose in the moderate range (5 to 6 Gy), whereas a dose of 2.5 Gy results in temporary sterility (12 months' duration).

Another potential hazard of testicular irradiation is the production of chromosome aberrations that may be passed on to succeeding generations. The fertile period occurring postexposure does not exclude the possibility of chromosome damage in functional spermatozoa. Chromosome changes in the immature spermatogonia also cannot be discounted, and may either be propagated or eliminated through the many divisions needed to produce spermatozoa.

Diagnostic Radiology and Nuclear Medicine.—These two clinical specialties involving acute low doses to patients and chronic low doses to personnel present no hazard in terms of sterility. These doses, however, may produce chromosomal changes, possibly resulting in mutations in future generations. For this reason, the utmost care should be taken to shield the testes from unnecessary radiation of all types.

Radiation Therapy.—In contrast to diagnostic procedures, total doses administered in radiotherapy can produce sterility in addition

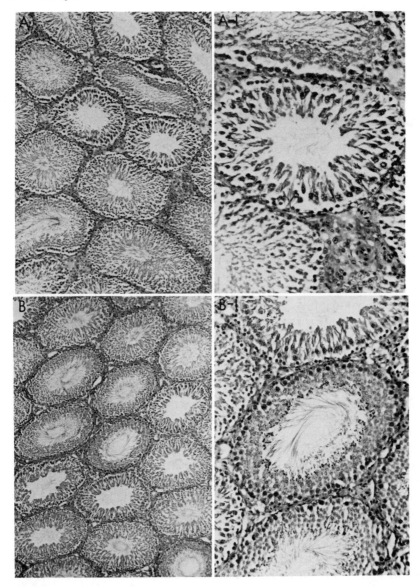

FIG 6–7.
Testes from a rat exposed to 5 Gy total body radiation. **A** and **A-1,** normal testes illustrating both immature and mature cell types. **B** and **B-1,** one week postexposure illustrating minimal changes; mature sperm are still present. *(Continued.)*

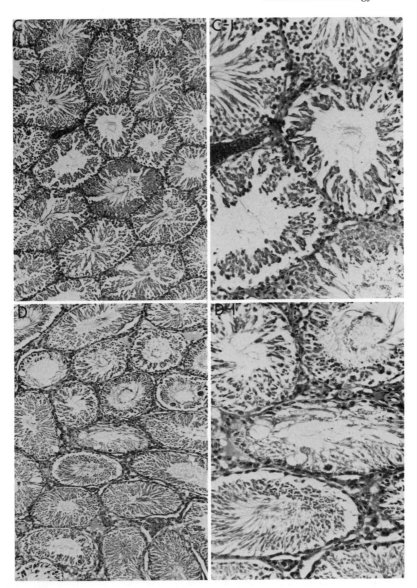

FIG 6–7 (cont.).
C and C-1, three weeks; D and D-1, four weeks postexposure; both times exhibit disap-
pearance of normal architecture, looseness in the appearance of the network, and a decrease
in all cells, both precursor and mature, with a loss of polarity in the remaining cells. (H & E
stain; A to D magnification × 100; A-1 to D-1 magnification × 250.)

to chromosomal changes. Every effort should be made to shield the testes from scattered radiation when the treatment field is situated close to this tissue. In addition, the patient should be informed of the possibility of temporary or permanent sterility and be given procreation advice when the situation warrants it. Another point that must be clarified is that impotency is not caused by radiation-induced sterility.

Female

The ova are contained within saclike enclosures (follicles), designated by size as small, intermediate, and large, which vary in radiosensitivity as follows: intermediate follicles, most sensitive; small follicles, most resistant, and mature follicles, moderately sensitive. Unlike in the male, the reproductive cells in the female are not constantly dividing and replacing those lost through menstruation. An ovum is released from a mature follicle at ovulation, followed by either fertilization or menstruation. An initial period of fertility occurs after moderate doses of radiation to the ovaries, due to the presence of moderately resistant mature follicles that can release an ovum. This fertile period is followed by temporary or permament sterility resulting from damage to ova in the radiosensitive intermediate follicles, which inhibits their maturation and release. Fertility may recur due to the maturation of ova in the radioresistant small follicles.

Although the dose necessary to produce sterility in females is a function of age (a higher dose is necessary in young women than in older women), in general, a dose of greater than 6.25 Gy produces sterility in women.

Major concern arises over the possibility of genetic changes in functional ova after irradiation. Although fertility recurs after low and moderate doses, the possibility cannot be excluded that these functional ova have incurred chromosome damage that may result in either grossly abnormal offspring or in offspring carrying nonvisible mutations that can be passed on to succeeding generations.

Diagnostic Radiology and Nuclear Medicine.—As in the male, low doses received from diagnostic procedures do not produce sterility in the female, but may cause chromosome changes. Although the body forms a natural shield for the ovaries, precautions always should be taken to avoid unnecessary ovarian exposure whenever possible.

Radiation Therapy.—Doses in the therapeutic range pose a double hazard: chromosomal damage and sterility. In addition, unlike in the male, where radiation-induced sterility does not produce effects in secondary sexual organs resulting in impotency, radiation sterilization of the female may produce an artificial menopause with marked effects on secondary genitalia and sexual characteristics. In the case of a malignant disease requiring irradiation of the ovaries, the patient should be informed of the possible consequences. Also, when sterility is not induced but the ovaries receive significant scattered radiation, procreation advice always should be given to the patient.

Eye

The lens of the eye contains a population of actively dividing cells that may be damaged and destroyed by radiation. Because there is no mechanism for removal of injured cells, those damaged cells form a cataract (a lens opacity). Moderate doses of radiation (as low as 2 Gy) produce cataracts in a few individuals, with the incidence increasing to 100% in individuals exposed to an acute dose of 7 Gy. The degree of opacity is reflected as visual impairment, ranging from minimal impairment at 2 Gy, becoming progressive, and causing complete visual obstruction at higher doses. The frequency of cataracts varies with exposure to chronic and acute doses, with chronic doses producing a lower frequency of cataracts than acute doses.

Diagnostic Radiology.—Because radiation is scattered to the eye during fluoroscopic procedures, occupationally exposed personnel may exhibit cataracts. More common in the early days of radiology when little knowledge existed of the biologic effects and hazards of radiation, cataracts are considered a late effect of radiation, appearing from 1 to 30 years postexposure (Chapter 8). Although doses in diagnostic radiology today are much lower and equipment is vastly improved, precautions should be taken to shield the eyes during fluoroscopic procedures.

Radiation Therapy.—Doses to the eye in the therapeutic range certainly can induce cataracts. The minimal cataract inducing dose appears to be a total of 4 Gy. Total doses of 12 Gy delivered by fractionated schedules induce cataracts in almost all patients, becoming progressive at 14 Gy. When treating lesions of the face located near the eyes, eye shields should always be used to reduce the formation and severity of cataracts.

CARDIOVASCULAR SYSTEM

Vasculature

Blood vessel damage may result in occlusion through two means: (1) damaged endothelial cells, or substances released from them, may stimulate division of undamaged cells in regenerative efforts (if too many cells are replaced, occlusion may occur); or (2) destruction of the endothelial cells may induce the formation of blood clots in the vessels (thrombosis). Small vessels, possibly due to their small lumens, are more radiosensitive than large vessels. These changes in blood vessels may be manifested in chronic changes such as petechial hemorrhages (pinpoint hemorrhages), telangiectasia (dilation of small terminal vessels), and vessel sclerosis (a type of fibrosis—actually, a hardening and concomitant loss of elasticity of the vessel wall).

Because blood vessels are responsible for the transport of oxygen and nutrients to all organs of the body, occlusion of the vessels can have serious consequences to any organ. A complete loss of oxygen and nutrients will result in necrosis of the cells and tissues of that organ. A partial loss of these substances may result in atrophy and fibrosis of the organ, with a corresponding decrease in functional ability and a generalized decreased ability to withstand trauma.

Heart

Although for many years the heart was believed to be radioresistant, closer appraisal of the response of the heart to radiation is throwing doubts on this thought. Although the heart is undamaged at low and moderate doses except for functional (EKG) changes, high doses can produce pericarditis (inflammation of the pericardium, the membrane covering the heart) and pancarditis (inflammation of the entire heart).

Diagnostic Radiology and Nuclear Medicine.—Doses in these two clinical areas are not of sufficient magnitude to produce changes in the heart.

Radiation Therapy.—The heart is often totally or partially included in the radiation field, e.g., in the treatment of malignant lymphomas and of the chest wall following mastectomy for breast cancer. Fractionated doses totaling 40 Gy produce the above changes in a small percentage of individuals, with the incidence increasing with increasing dose. When possible, the heart should be shielded during the entire treatment course, and particularly when total doses exceed 40 Gy.

GROWING BONE AND CARTILAGE

Although mature bone and cartilage are radioresistant, growing bone and cartilage are moderately radiosensitive. In general, mature bone is formed through the mineralization (calcium deposition) of cartilage. Growing bone and cartilage consist of both nondividing, differentiated cells (osteocytes, chondrocytes) and rapidly dividing, undifferentiated cells (osteoblasts, chondroblasts); the latter group accounts for the moderate sensitivity of these tissues.

Damage to both small blood vessels and bone marrow also plays an important contributing role in radiation injury to growing bone. Moderate doses of radiation produce temporary inhibition of mitosis and death of the proliferating immature cells. Recovery does occur at doses of this magnitude, resulting in minimal late damage.

High doses may produce a permanent inhibition of mitosis and destruction of proliferating cells, resulting in cessation of bone formation. Few early gross changes are evident in bone even at these high doses. However, alterations in shape and size of the bone and scoliosis are evident late changes.

Diagnostic Radiology and Nuclear Medicine.—The low doses administered during these procedures do not result in the changes outlined above. However, the administration of bone-seeking radionuclides can cause these changes.

Radiation Therapy.—Treatment of Wilms' tumor and neuroblastoma in children often unavoidably includes a growing bone in the radiation field, therefore producing bone abnormalities and scoliosis. Fractionated total doses greater than 20 Gy produce marked changes in the bones of children irradiated when less than 2 years of age. The incidence of bone abnormalities decreases with decreasing dose and increasing age at time of treatment.

LIVER

The liver is usually considered part of the digestive system (an accessory gland essential to storage, metabolism and excretion of the products of the digestive process). For many years the liver was considered to be radioresistant, but current opinion is that the liver is a moderately sensitive, responsive organ.

The hepatic cells (parenchymal cells of the liver), while relatively resistant to radiation, do retain the capability of regeneration through mitosis. However, the liver has a large blood supply and a great number of both large and small blood vessels; for this reason, radiation injury to the hepatic cells is believed to be secondary to vascular changes.

Low and moderate doses produce little observable acute response; early changes after high doses are difficult to detect, except possibly through function studies. In some cases, the liver may be enlarged and fluid may accumulate in the abdominal cavity (ascites).

Delayed radiation effects in the liver, termed *radiation hepatitis*, are a consequence of vascular sclerosis and consist primarily of fibrosis (sometimes called *cirrhosis*). The primary lesion observed in the human liver after irradiation is veno-occlusive disease, which impairs the function of the liver, resulting in liver failure and jaundice.

Diagnostic Radiology and Nuclear Medicine.—No observable response is detected in the liver subsequent to the doses delivered by these procedures.

Radiation Therapy.—The liver, either totally or partially, is sometimes included in the treatment field, e.g., in the treatment of malignant diseases of the kidney, lymphomas, and ovarian cancer with moving-strip or whole-abdomen technique. Doses in the clinical range produce radiation hepatitis, ranging from 35 to 45 Gy with a standard fractionation schedule. The clinical significance of this will depend on the volume of the organ irradiated.

RESPIRATORY SYSTEM

The respiratory system consists of the nose, pharynx, trachea, and lungs. Although considered relatively resistant to radiation, the lungs are actually responsive to radiation in the high dose range (greater than a single dose of 10 Gy).

The primary early change in the lungs after irradiation is inflammation, termed *radiation pneumonitis*. This is a transitory response after moderate doses, and recovery occurs with minimal damage. A high dose to both lungs produces a progressive reaction that may develop from an early pneumonitis to chronic fibrosis, an outcome that can certainly cause death (Fig 6–8).

Diagnostic Radiology and Nuclear Medicine.—Radiation pneumonitis is not a response observed in the lungs after low doses.

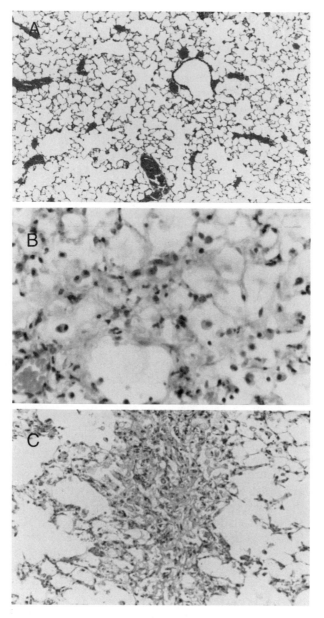

FIG 6–8.
Lungs from an unirradiated mouse (**A**); 20 weeks after 13 Gy ($\sim LD_{50}$) (**B**); and at 52 weeks
after a sublethal dose of 11 Gy (**C**). The acute response seen in **B** is termed *radiation
pneumonitis* and occurs between 3 and 7 months after radiation, whereas the late fibrotic
response in **C** occurs 9 months after radiation. Pneumonitis is characterized by edema and
cellular infiltrate, whereas the fibrotic response is a focal scarring process with the laying
down of collagen.

Radiation Therapy.—One lung is often the primary treatment area, or a portion of it may be included in the treatment field when other organs are irradiated, e.g., irradiation of the breast. Doses of 25 Gy to both lungs with a standard fractionation schedule may produce a progressive fibrosis in a small percentage (8%) of individuals treated. Increasing doses cause corresponding increases in the numbers of patients with this response, reaching 50% at a total dose of 30 Gy. The response is dependent on the volume irradiated; one lung can be given a higher dose than both lungs. Although fibrosis occurs in the irradiated lung, rendering it nonfunctional, the remaining, undamaged lung continues to function.

URINARY SYSTEM

The kidneys, ureters, bladder, and urethra constitute the urinary system. Damage in the kidney, termed *radiation nephritis*, appears as a loss of tubules (Fig 6–9), with little change in the glomeruli. The kidney becomes atrophic and renal failure ensues.

Work on the bladder by Stewart and her colleagues has shown that damage in the bladder of experimental mice does not occur before 6 months after large single doses, with the maximum damage expressed at 1 year after all doses. The major pathologic changes were epithelial denudation and loss of the specialized surface cells of the bladder. Fibrosis of the muscularis did not appear until after 12 months.

Diagnostic Radiology and Nuclear Medicine.—Doses from diagnostic radiography, fluoroscopy, and nuclear medicine do not produce this response in the urinary system.

Radiation Therapy.—When both kidneys are included in the treatment field, they must be shielded at a total dose of 26 Gy. The statistical incidence of these changes occurring increases sharply after this dose—28 Gy to both kidneys in 5 weeks results in a high probability of fatal radiation nephritis.

As in the lungs, the volume irradiated plays an important role. Exclusion of one third of the kidney volume from the treatment field greatly minimizes renal failure. When irradiation is given to only one kidney, the unirradiated kidney will continue to function if the irradiated one is surgically resected.

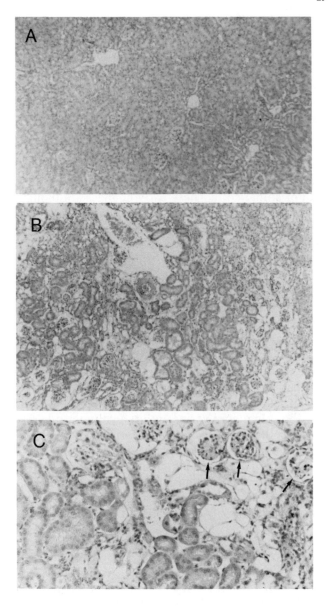

FIG 6–9.
Histologic sections of kidney from a nonirradiated mouse (**A**) and a low-power view (**B**) and higher-power view (**C**) from an irradiated mouse. Note the empty holes in the kidney of the irradiated mouse, representing a loss of tubules. **C** shows glomeruli *(arrows)*, which are surrounded by once existent but now destroyed tubules.

CENTRAL NERVOUS SYSTEM

The nervous system consists of the brain and spinal cord. In general, the cells of the various parts of the nervous system are nondividing differentiated cells, rendering them relatively radioresistant. In fact, the nervous system is considered the most radioresistant system in the adult; therefore, low and moderate doses of radiation will result in minimal, if any, morphologic damage (however, some authors have reported functional changes at low doses).

Early changes in the CNS after high doses include inflammation (termed *myelitis* in the spinal cord), progressing to necrosis and fibrosis of the brain or spinal cord. These early changes are thought to be due to loss of glial cells, whereas the chronic changes are suggested to be of vascular origin. Of particular interest is the comparatively higher radiosensitivity of the white than the gray matter of the brain. The threshold level for radiation injury to the CNS is between 20 and 40 Gy.

Diagnostic Radiology and Nuclear Medicine.—No observable changes result from doses of this low magnitude.

Radiation Therapy.—Doses in the clinical range totaling 50 Gy can cause delayed radiation necrosis in the brain. Because brain irradiation occurs for treatment of brain tumors, it is often difficult to distinguish the effects caused by the tumor from those caused by irradiation. The response of the spinal cord varies with the volume and area irradiated; the cervical and thoracic cord are both more sensitive than the lumbar cord. The incidence of radiation myelitis increases at doses greater than 50 Gy given to small volumes and greater than 45 Gy to large volumes. This is of importance because the cord is often included in the treatment field of many diseases, e.g., lung cancer, cancer of the esophagus, Hodgkin's disease, and tumors of the head and neck region.

REFERENCES

1. Anderson WAD: *Pathology*, ed 6. St. Louis, CV Mosby, 1971.
2. Berdjis CC: *Pathology of Irradiation*. Baltimore, Williams & Wilkins, 1971.
3. Casarett AP: *Radiation Biology*. Englewood Cliffs, NJ, Prentice-Hall, 1968.
4. Fletcher GH: *Textbook of Radiotherapy*, ed 3. Philadelphia, Lea & Febiger, 1980.

5. Moss W, et al: *Radiation Oncology: Rationale, Technique, Results,* ed 4. St Louis, CV Mosby, 1973.
6. Robbins SL: *Pathologic Basis of Disease.* Philadelphia, WB Saunders, 1974.
7. Rubin P, Casarett GW: *Clinical Radiation Pathology,* vols. I and II. Philadelphia, WB Saunders, 1968.
8. Stewart FA, Michael BD, Denekamp J: Late radiation damage in the mouse bladder as measured by increased urination frequency. *Radiat Res* 1978; 75:649–659.
9. Travis EL: Relative radiosensitivity of the human lung. *Adv Radiat Biol* 1987; 12:205–238.
10. van der Kogel AJ: *Late Effects of Radiation on the Spinal Cord: Dose-Effect Relationships and Pathogenesis* (dissertation). Publication of the Radiobiological Institute of the Organization for Health Research TNO, Rijswijk, The Netherlands, 1979.
11. Withers HR, Mason KA, Thames HD Jr: Late radiation response of kidney assayed by tubule cell survival. *Br J Radiol* 1986; 59:587–595.

Chapter 7 _____

Total Body Radiation Response

_____

The response of the organism to total body irradiation is determined by the combined response of all systems in the body. Because systems differ in their radiosensitivities and, therefore, their responses (Chapters 4 and 6), the total body response will be a function of the particular system most affected by the radiation. The previous two chapters dealt with the responses of specific organs and systems to radiation; these findings will now be applied to the response of the organism to acute total body radiation, in both adult and fetal life.

ADULT

The response of an adult organism to an acute total body exposure to radiation results in specific signs, symptoms, and clinical findings. The relationship of these signs and symptoms to a specific type of trauma or disease process is termed a *syndrome*. Because the response of the organism to total body radiation results in specific findings, the term "total body syndrome" or "radiation syndrome" is used. Although damage to one particular system is responsible for the syndrome, the manifestation of the specific signs and symptoms is a result of damage to more than one system in the body.

Radiation Syndrome in Mammals

"Total body radiation syndrome" applies only when exposure occurs under a specific set of conditions. First, exposure of the organism must have occurred acutely—to be more exact—in a matter of minutes, rather than hours or days. Second, the area of the organism exposed to radiation must be total-body, or very nearly total-body, to manifest the full-blown radiation syndrome. Third, the radiation syndromes are produced by exposure to external penetrating sources such as x-rays, γ-rays, and neutrons; radioactive materials deposited internally do not induce the full syndrome.

Survival Time.—The primary effect of an acute total body radiation exposure is to shorten the life span of the organism, the degree of which is dependent on the dose to which an organism is exposed. Because the life span of an organism is drastically reduced after a moderate to high dose of total body radiation (after exposure the organism may live as long as 1 to 2 months or only hours), total body exposures in this dose range are considered immediately lethal.

The survival time of an organism exposed to total body radiation is expressed as the mean (average) survival time. Variations in survival time exist among different species and even among animals within the same species. Some animals live longer than others due to these individual variations in sensitivity. The expression of survival time as the mean takes these variations into account, therefore eliminating those individuals who appear to be extremely radiosensitive or radioresistant.

TABLE 7–1.

LD$_{50/30}$ Values for Different Species

Species	LD$_{50/30}$* (Gy)
Human	2.5–3.0
Monkey	4.0
Dog	3.0
Rabbit	8.0
Rat	9.0
Mouse	9.0
Chicken	6.0
Frog	7.0
Goldfish	20.0

*In humans the expression LD$_{50/60}$ may be more useful (for explanation, see the text). In addition, this figure is an estimate based on the small number of accidental overexposures; more data may change these estimates.

In this way a general pattern of survival time will appear when large numbers of animals are irradiated.

Because of the variations in survival time of a group of animals exposed to the same total body dose, the relationship of survival time of an entire population of the same species (e.g., all dogs or all monkeys) exposed to the same total body dose is expressed as that dose which kills a certain percentage of the population within a given period of time. For example, the lethal dose necessary to kill 50% of a population in 30 days is expressed as the LD$_{50/30}$ dose; the lethal dose necessary to kill 100% of the population in 6 days is the LD$_{100/6}$ dose. The LD$_{50/30}$ dose is the most often-used expression when discussing total body exposures, although in humans the LD$_{50/60}$ dose is more relevant. The reasons for this will be discussed in a later section. Table 7–1 lists the LD$_{50/30}$ doses in Gy for different species.

Dose and Survival Time.—A curve can be constructed relating survival time to dose for all mammals exposed to total body radiation (Fig 7–1). As dose increases, the number of survivors and survival time decrease accordingly. At a dose of approximately 2 Gy, death will occur in a small percentage of the animals, the percentage increasing with increasing dose. In this dose range, survival time is dose-dependent, i.e., decreasing with increasing dose. Mean survival time does not appear to be a function of dose between 10 and 100 Gy. All animals irradiated with a total body dose in this range survive for approximately the same length of time. However, fewer animals survive these doses than the lower doses. Mean survival time becomes dose-dependent (decreases with increasing dose) at doses of 100 Gy and over; in addition, the number of survivors decreases.

The three general regions of the curve in Figure 7–1 reflect damage to three different systems that may result in the death of the animal. This does not indicate that other organs and systems have not sustained radiation damage, but rather that the primary cause of death is destruction of one specific system. The three defined radiation syndromes are based on the failed organ system responsible for death.

At doses between 1 and 10 Gy, death occurs, primarily as a result of damage to the hemopoietic system, in particular, to destruction of the bone marrow. The total body syndrome reflected in this dose range is termed the *hemopoietic* or the *bone marrow syndrome.*

In the second region of the dose response curve (10 to 100 Gy), death is primarily due to damage in the gastrointestinal (GI) system, particularly in the small intestine. The syndrome reflected in this dose range is the *GI syndrome.*

Doses greater than 100 Gy comprise the third area of the curve and

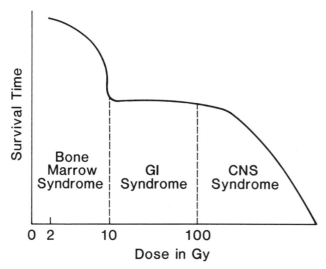

FIG 7–1.
Curve derived from studies of the response of different species to total body irradiation. Note the three distinct variations in survival time in the dose ranges of 2 to 10 Gy, 10 to 100 Gy, and >100 Gy, reflecting damage to the specific organ system for which the radiation syndromes are named. (From Pizzarello DJ, Witcofski RL:*Basic Radiation Biology.* Philadelphia, Lea & Febiger, 1967. Used by permission.)

reflect damage in the central nervous system (CNS). Because damage in this system is responsible for the death of the animal, the syndrome is referred to as the *CNS syndrome.*

Two points must be kept in mind concerning the generalized curve in Figure 7–1. First, the dose ranges given for each syndrome are not specific for humans; these figures are derived from studies of the responses of many different animals following acute total body exposure. Second, there is an overlap of the syndromes at the higher doses of each dose range (e.g., between 6 and 10 Gy some animals die from a combination of damage in the hemopoietic *and* GI systems). Therefore, the *threshold* for the GI syndrome may be 6 Gy. However, because the majority of animals die primarily from destruction of the GI tract after a dose of 10 Gy, the GI syndrome is associated with doses between 10 and 100 Gy. This same reasoning applies to the CNS syndrome. Doses less than 100 Gy will cause death from CNS damage in some animals, but the majority of animals die primarily from CNS destruction at doses greater than 100 Gy. Therefore, the threshold for the CNS syndrome is lower than 100 Gy, despite the fact that the syndrome is defined at this dose.

Stages of Response.—The response of an animal to an acute total body dose of radiation can be divided into three stages. The duration of each stage is dose-dependent (i.e., the lower the dose, the longer the duration of any of the three stages). Each stage may last from a period of weeks (low doses) to a matter of minutes (high doses).

The first phase is the *prodromal stage,* which is characterized by nausea, vomiting, and diarrhea (often referred to as the N-V-D syndrome). The prodromal stage may last from a few minutes to a few days, depending on the dose (the higher the dose, the shorter the prodromal stage).

The second phase is the *latent stage;* the term is derived from the generally healthy appearance of the animal during this time. However, changes are taking place in the respective systems damaged by the radiation that will eventually lead to either the demise or recovery of the animal. The duration of the latent stage varies with dose, from weeks at doses below 5 Gy, to hours or shorter at doses greater than 100 Gy.

After this time the animal becomes obviously ill and exhibits the specific signs and symptoms of the particular syndrome reflecting the organ system damaged. This third phase is termed, appropriately, the *manifest illness stage* and may last from minutes to weeks, depending on the dose. Finally, the animal either recovers or dies as a result of radiation injury. Table 7–2 summarizes these stages.

TABLE 7–2.

Stages of the Total-Body Syndrome

Stage	Duration	Major Symptoms
Prodromal	Days–minutes	N-V-D syndrome Nausea Vomiting Diarrhea
Latent	Weeks–hours	None
Manifest illness	Weeks–hours	Symptoms reflect the systems damaged: Bone marrow—fever, malaise Gastrointestinal—malaise, anorexia, severe diarrhea, fever, dehydration, electrolyte imbalance CNS—lethargy, tremors, convulsions, nervousness, watery diarrhea, coma

The three radiation syndromes will be discussed in relation to findings in humans. Although the time of appearance of the signs and symptoms varies among different mammals, generally speaking, all mammals will exhibit similar signs and symptoms. Survival time following different doses varies greatly among species, with humans appearing to be a relatively radiosensitive species (see Table 7–1).

Radiation Syndrome in Humans

Data concerning the exposure of humans to acute total body radiation has been accumulated from the following sources:

1. Accidents in industry and laboratories (approximately 50 reported cases).
2. Pacific Testing Grounds accidents involving exposure to fallout.
3. The exposure of individuals at Hiroshima and Nagasaki.
4. Medical exposures involving total-body or near total-body radiation for cancer therapy or other reasons.
5. The nuclear accident at Chernobyl in the Soviet Union.

Although all of these situations provide an opportunity to study the response of humans to total body radiation, difficulties arise over the estimation of dose and the extent of exposure received by individuals in all cases except, possibly, one: medical exposure. In spite of these problems, the study of these individuals has identified a general pattern of the radiation syndromes in humans. One important point to keep in mind is that in most of these individuals, medical support resulted in an increased survival time. Without this life-sustaining support, survival time would be decreased.

Bone Marrow Syndrome.—The bone marrow syndrome in humans occurs after doses between 1 and 10 Gy, with death occurring in a few individuals at a dose of 2 Gy. The $LD_{50/60}$* for humans is approximately 2.5 to 3.0 Gy and is in the dose range of the bone marrow syndrome. Death of the individual is due to destruction of the bone marrow to an extent that will not support life.

The prodromal stage of the bone marrow syndrome occurs a few hours postexposure and consists mainly of nausea and vomiting. The latent stage lasts from a few days to 3 weeks postexposure, during which time the number of cells in the circulating blood is not severely depressed. The individual appears and feels well during this time; however, stem cells in the bone marrow are dying during both the prodromal and the latent stages, resulting in a decreased production of mature cells and, therefore, a decrease in the number of cells in the circulating blood. This drop in blood cell count appears during the manifest illness stage, beginning at 3 weeks and possibly continuing through the 5th week postexposure (at low doses). During this time the individual exhibits the specific signs and symptoms of the bone marrow syndrome. The depression of all blood cell counts (pancytopenia) results in anemia and hemorrhage (due to depression of RBCs) and serious infections (due to the depression of white cells—leukopenia).

Survival in the radiation dose range of the bone marrow syndrome decreases with increasing dose. At the lower limits of the dose range, 1 to 3 Gy, bone marrow cells will repopulate the marrow to an extent great enough to support life in the majority of individuals (Fig 7–2). Full recovery of a large percentage of these individuals will occur from 3 weeks to 6 months postexposure. A few sensitive individuals may die 6 to 8 weeks after an exposure of 2 Gy; doses from 4 to 6 Gy (dose range of the $LD_{50/60}$) result in a decreased number of survivors. In these individuals partial repopulation of the bone marrow may occur, but not to a sufficient extent to support life. No human has been reported as surviving a dose of 10 Gy.

As dose increases, survival time decreases, death occurring in ap-

---

*Because humans appear to both develop and recover from the bone marrow syndrome later than other species, deaths may occur as late as 60 days postexposure. In addition, the majority of deaths occur by 30 days in humans, whereas in animals they occur by 15 days. For these reasons, the expression $LD_{50/60}$ may be more meaningful in humans than the $LD_{50/30}$ used in animals.

proximately 4 to 6 weeks after doses of 3 to 5 Gy, but in 2 weeks at doses of 5 to 10 Gy.

The primary cause of death in the bone marrow syndrome is destruction of the bone marrow, resulting in infection and hemorrhage. The bone marrow is normally filled with cells that supply mature cells to the circulating blood. After exposures in this dose range, the number of cells in the bone marrow steadily decreases until the bone marrow

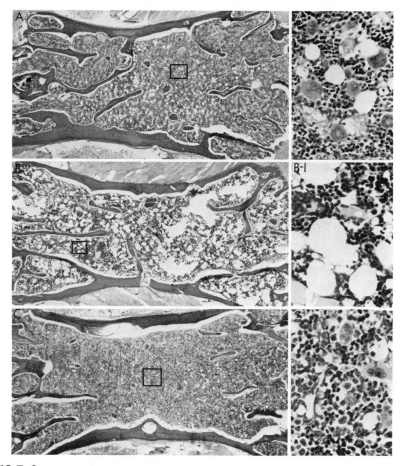

FIG 7–2.
Rat bone marrow following a total body dose of 5 Gy. **A,** normal. **B,** one week postexposure exhibiting hypocellularity and relative increase in fat. **C,** three weeks postexposure, contents now appear relatively normal, indicating regeneration (absence of bony trabeculae in **C** is not a result of irradiation but is due to the area of the tissue sectioned). (H & E stain; A to C magnification × 40; A-1 to C-1 magnification × 300.)

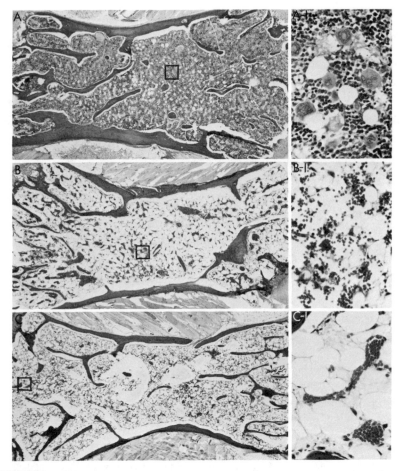

FIG 7–3.
Rat bone marrow following a total body dose of 10 Gy (**B** and **B-1**) and 20 Gy (**C** and **C-1**), both illustrating a dramatic hypocellularity and increased fat content compared with normal marrow (**A** and **A-1**). Those cells present are red blood cells due to hemorrhage. (H & E stain; A to C magnification × 40; A–1 to C–1 magnification × 300.)

is not capable of producing the cells that are necessary in the circulating blood to sustain life (Fig 7–3).

Survival after whole body doses in the range of the bone marrow syndrome can be improved by transplanting bone marrow from a matched histocompatible donor to the irradiated individual. Bone marrow transplantation has proved to be of some limited use in treating victims of nuclear accidents who received sufficiently high doses to die of this syndrome. At Chernobyl, of the 50 patients who received more than 5 Gy, a lethal dose, 21 (42%) survived after receiving bone marrow transplants. Thus, at least some victims can benefit from advanced hematologic care.

GI Syndrome.—The second defined acute radiation syndrome is the GI syndrome. Doses between 10 and 100 Gy will result in the GI syndrome in all animals studied; however, in humans, some symptoms of the GI syndrome appear after a dose of 6 Gy (the threshold dose). The full syndrome is apparent after 10 Gy. The LD_{100} for humans (between 6 and 10 Gy) is within the dose range of the GI syndrome. Survival time does not vary with dose in this syndrome; death occurs at the same time, regardless of dose. In humans, death occurs within 3 to 10 days if medical support is not administered, and within approximately 2 weeks even with medical support.

The prodromal stage of the GI syndrome occurs within a few hours postexposure and is characterized by severe nausea and vomiting, which may be accompanied by severe cramps and diarrhea. From the 2nd through the 5th day, the individual enters the latent stage and feels well. At the end of this time, there is a recurrence of severe diarrhea, nausea, and vomiting accompanied by fever, signaling the onset of the manifest illness stage, which may persist from the 5th through the 10th day. Death occurs from the GI syndrome during the 2nd week postexposure if life-sustaining support has been administered (fluids, transfusions, etc).

The GI syndrome is due to damage in two organ systems: the GI tract and the bone marrow. The full GI syndrome does not occur if only the GI tract has been irradiated, because the bone marrow plays an integral role in this syndrome.

The lining of the GI tract, particularly the small intestine, is severely damaged by doses in this range. The mitotic activity of the cells in the crypts of Lieberkühn, the radiosensitive precursor cells to the population of cells on the villi, is decreased drastically following exposure. As a result, the villi, which slough dead cells into the intestinal lumen every 24 hours and are dependent on the crypts of Lieberkühn for replacements, lose cells and become shortened, flattened, and partially or completely denuded (Figs 7–4 and 7–5).

The consequences to the individual of these changes in the GI tract are profound. The flattened villi result in decreased absorption of materials across the intestinal wall. Fluids leak into the lumen of the GI tract, resulting in dehydration. Overwhelming infection occurs as bacteria that normally live within the GI tract gain access to the bloodstream through the intestinal wall causing systemic infection.

The effects of these drastic changes in the GI tract are compounded by equally drastic changes in the bone marrow. In fact, the effects of damage in the bone marrow occur at a time when damage in the GI tract is reaching its maximum. Of primary importance is the severe decrease in the number of circulating white cells. This depression occurs as bacteria are invading the bloodstream from the GI tract, therefore compounding an already severe problem. The numbers of remaining blood cells may not severely decrease because death occurs before radiation damage is reflected in these cell lines.

Although attempts at regeneration occur in the GI tract after irradiation, particularly after the lower doses associated with the GI syndrome, the damage incurred by the bone marrow will probably still result in death (Fig 7–6). Death from the GI syndrome is due primarily to infection, dehydration, and electrolyte imbalance resulting from the destructive and irreparable changes in the GI tract and bone marrow.

It is estimated that 22 victims of the Chernobyl nuclear accident in the Soviet Union received total body doses between 6 and 16 Gy, which is within the range of the GI syndrome. Nineteen of these victims died within 4 to 15 days, the time when death from the GI syndrome occurs.

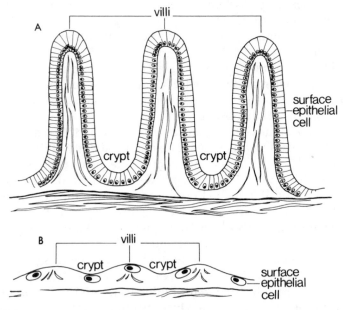

FIG 7–4.
Diagrammatic representation of changes in the small intestine following total body exposure in the dose range of the GI syndrome. **A,** preirradiation; **B,** postirradiation.

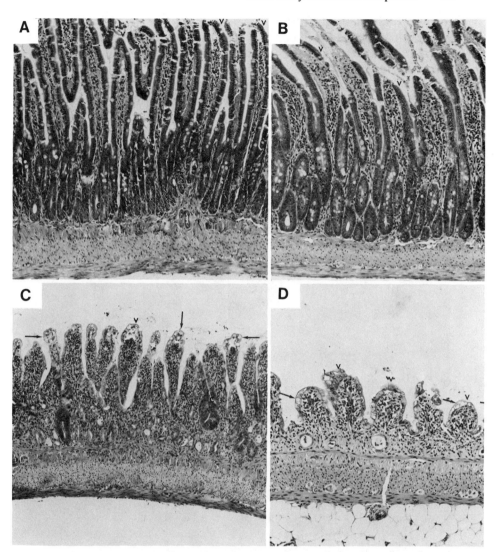

FIG 7–5.
Small intestine of rats following various doses of total body irradiation, all sacrificed 5 days postexposure. **A,** normal; note villi *(V)* and crypts *(C)*. **B,** 5 Gy; minimal shortening and sloughing of cells from villi is evident. **C,** 10 Gy; blunted villi with atypical epithelial cells *(arrows);* crypts contain mitotic figures. **D,** 20 Gy; absence of crypts; sloughing and edema of villi. Note atypical changes in epithelial cells at this dose *(arrows).* (H & E stain, magnification × 75.)

However, skin damage from thermal burns in these patients was in itself sufficiently severe to be life-threatening. Since death from the GI syndrome is due to damage not only to the gut but also to the bone marrow, bone marrow transplants could be useful in these individuals. The experience at Chernobyl indicates that although bone marrow transplantation could be useful in saving some individuals who received less than 10 Gy, bone marrow transplantation has little effect after total body doses greater than 10 Gy. After these doses, depletion of jejunal crypt cells is so extensive that adequate repopulation and restoration of the intestinal mucosa cannot occur.

CNS Syndrome.—The full CNS syndrome occurs after doses of greater than 50 Gy in humans. Although CNS damage is evident at lower doses (20 Gy), death from the full CNS syndrome occurs within 2 to 3 days following an exposure of 50 Gy in all individuals.

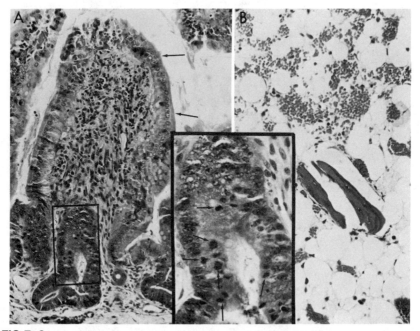

FIG 7–6.
GI tract and bone marrow of rat exposed to 10 Gy total body irradiation. **A,** high-power view of edematous villi exhibiting atypical epithelial cells *(arrows)* and crypt with numerous mitotic figures. **Inset** indicates regenerative attempts *(arrows)*. **B,** bone marrow from same animal. Note the absence of all stem cells; only red blood cells are present. Although regenerative efforts occur in the crypts, the damage in the bone marrow is sufficient to cause death of the animal. (H & E stain; A and B magnification × .175; insert magnification × 350.)

The prodromal stage varies from a few minutes to a few hours dependent on dose. The signs and symptoms of this phase are extreme nervousness, confusion, severe nausea and vomiting, a loss of consciousness, and complaints of burning sensations of the skin. A latent period next appears and may last for several hours, although often it is of shorter duration. The manifest illness stage begins 5 to 6 hours postexposure, at which time there is a return of watery diarrhea, convulsions, coma, and finally death.

The cause of death in the CNS syndrome is not fully known or understood. Examination of the CNS after an individual has been exposed to a dose within this range reveals few changes in the parenchymal cells of the brain. This is not surprising, as these cells are nondividing and do not manifest damage as do the cells in the bone marrow or the GI tract, in which division of stem cells is necessary to provide the end cell to carry on function. Damage in the CNS may be a result of damage to the blood vessels that supply the system, resulting in edema in the cranial vault, vasculitis (inflammatory changes in the vessels), and meningitis (inflammation of the meninges). Death is suggested to be due to increased pressure in the confining cranial vault as a result of increased fluid content caused by these changes.

The bone marrow and the GI tract do not exhibit dramatic changes in the CNS syndrome because the individual does not live long enough. An increased survival time would result in the manifestation of dramatic changes in these systems.

The three radiation syndromes described above are outlined in Table 7–3.

EMBRYO AND FETUS

Radiation has long been known to have profoundly damaging effects on the developing embryo. For obvious reasons, systematic studies of the effects of radiation on the developing embryo have been conducted in laboratory animals, particularly mice and rats. These studies have resulted in a wealth of information on this subject, including the definition of specific effects induced by radiation.

There are three general effects of radiation on the embryo and fetus:

1. Lethality.
2. Congenital abnormalities present at birth.
3. Long-term effects (late effects) that are not visible at birth but develop later in life.

TABLE 7–3.

Summary of Acute Radiation Syndromes in Humans After Whole-Body Irradiation*

Syndrome	Dose Range	Time of Death	Organ and System Damaged	Signs and Symptoms Findings	Recovery Time
Hemopoietic	1–10 Gy[††]	3 wks–2 mos	Bone marrow	Decreased number of stem cells in bone marrow, increased amount of fat in bone marrow, pancytopenia, anemia, hemorrhage, infection	Dose dependent, 3 wks to 6 mos; some individuals do not survive
GI	10–50 Gy[‡]	3–10 days	Small intestine	Denudation of villi in small intestine, neutropenia, infection, bone marrow depression, electrolyte imbalance, watery diarrhea	None
CNS	>50 Gy	<3 days	Brain	Vasculitis, edema, meningitis	None

*From Rubin P, Casarett GW: *Clinical Radiation Pathology*, vol II. Philadelphia, WB Saunders Co, 1968. Used by permission.
†LD$_{50/60}$ for humans in this dose range (2.5–3.0 Gy).
‡LD$_{100}$ for humans in this dose range (10 Gy).

These effects can be produced in the embryo and fetus by a mutation in the ovum or sperm resulting in inherited (genetic) effects, or they can be directly induced by exposure of the fetus to radiation (congenital).

This section will discuss only those effects induced by irradiation in utero (congenital effects). In addition, the discussion will be limited to radiation-induced lethal effects and congenital abnormalities present at birth or shortly thereafter. Late effects will be discussed in a subsequent chapter. Because laboratory animals have been the primary source of information concerning this topic, the effects discussed will be those observed in these animals, unless otherwise stated. The extrapolation and implication of these findings for humans and observations in humans are presented at the end of this chapter.

Fetal Development

Radiation-induced lethality and specific gross abnormalities in the embryo and fetus are dependent on the day of gestation (in fact, the *part of day* of gestation) at which exposure occurs. For this reason, a basic knowledge of fetal development will give the reader a better understanding of radiation effects.

Russell and Russell have divided fetal development into three general stages: *pre-implantation, major organogenesis,* and *fetal* (growth) *stage*. In humans, the *pre-implantation stage* occurs from conception to 10 days postconception and precedes implantation of the embryo in the uterine wall. During this time the fertilized ovum repeatedly divides, forming a ball of cells that are highly undifferentiated.

Implantation of this ball of cells (the embryo) in the uterine wall signals the onset of the second stage, *major organogenesis,* which extends through the 6th week postconception in humans. During this time the cells of the embryo begin differentiating into the various stem cells that eventually will form all the organs of the body. The initial differentiation of cells to form a certain organ occurs on a specific gestational day. In humans, for example, neuroblasts (stem cells of the CNS) appear on the 18th gestational day, the forebrain and eyes begin to form on the 20th day, and on the 21st day the primitive germ cells appear.

At the end of the 6th week postconception, the embryo is termed a fetus and enters the *fetal stage,* primarily a period of growth. The fetus at this time contains most organ systems and many types of cells, ranging from undifferentiated stem cells to more differentiated cells.

Further attention should be given the development of the CNS. In adults, the CNS consists primarily of nondividing highly differentiated cells; the fetal CNS is in direct contrast to this. The neuroblasts appear at a very early point in fetal development (in humans on the 18th day) and are the most abundant and scattered cells present at all stages of embryonic development. As development progresses and the fetus grows in size, the neuroblasts become more diffusely dispersed throughout the body, in addition to undergoing some differentiation and becoming less mitotically active. However, the majority of these cells continue to exist throughout fetal development and until at least 2 weeks after birth. In fact, complete development of the CNS in humans may not occur until 10 to 12 years of age.

Based on the characteristics of fetal development and the fact that radiosensitivity is related to mitotic activity and differentiation, the fetus can be expected to be highly vulnerable not only to the lethal effects of radiation, but also to the induction of gross abnormalities recognizable at birth. After conception, one cell, the fertilized ovum, repeatedly divides and differentiates, producing the millions of various cells in the newborn animal. It is not surprising, then, that the developing embryo and fetus is exquisitely sensitive to radiation.

Radiation Effects on Fetal Development in Rodents

Pre-Implantation.—The effects of radiation on the embryo and fetus are a function of the stage of development during which exposure occurs. Figure 7–7 illustrates the effects of 2 Gy on mouse embryos exposed on different gestation days. The early embryo during pre-implantation and major organogenesis is exquisitely sensitive to ionizing radiation. Exposure during the pre-implantation stage results in a high incidence of prenatal deaths (death of the embryo before birth). This is not surprising, because the embryo consists of relatively few cells at this time; therefore, damage to one cell, the progenitor of many descendant cells, has a high probability of being fatal. Doses as low as 0.1 Gy have been reported fatal to the mouse embryo during this time. Those embryos that do survive exhibit few congenital abnormalities at birth; one specific abnormality that has been reported as a result of irradiation during pre-implantation is exencephaly (brain hernia, or protrusion of the brain through the top of the skull).

Major Organogenesis.—The incidence of congenital abnormalities in mouse embryos increases dramatically when exposure occurs during major organogenesis. Gross abnormalities have been observed in the

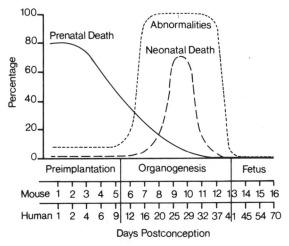

FIG 7–7.
Relationship of 2.0 Gy in utero exposure on different gestational days to the induction of lethality and major abnormalities in the mouse embryo. Lower scale indicates Rugh's time estimates for the three stages in the human embryo. (From Russell LB, Russell WL: An analysis of the changing radiation response of the developing mouse embryo. *J Cell Physiol* 1954; 1(suppl 43):103. Used by permission.)

mouse embryo exposed to 0.25 Gy during this stage. This is also the stage during which rubella (German measles) and the drug thalidomide are believed to wreak havoc on the fetus.

Although all major organs are beginning to form during this time, differentiation of cells to form various organs begins on specific days. As a result, irradiation on certain gestational days will result in specific abnormalities. For example, exposure of the mouse embryo on the 9th day results in a high incidence of ear and nose abnormalities, whereas exposure on the 10th day results in bone abnormalities. The greatest variety of congenital abnormalities is produced when radiation is given during the 8th to the 12th day in the mouse, corresponding to the 23rd to 37th day in humans. The time in which these abnormalities are produced is short, appearing to be when the cells initially differentiate and assume characteristics of the developing organ.

The majority of the effects of radiation on the fetus during this period of development are manifested in the CNS and in related sense organs, such as the eye. The sensitivity of the CNS is related to the abundance and immature characteristics of neuroblasts. Unlike cells in the adult, where the majority of cells in the CNS are nondividing, highly differentiated, and radioresistant, the neuroblasts in the fetus are highly undifferentiated, actively mitotic radiosensitive cells. These cells are scattered throughout the fetus, resulting in a high incidence of abnormalities involving the neurologic system. Some of the most common abnormalities of the CNS observed in mice after in utero irradiation include brain abnormalities such as microcephaly (small brain), hydrocephaly (water on the brain), and eye deformities such as microphthalmia (small eyes). Behavioral abnormalities such as mental retardation have been reported in humans.

The developing musculoskeletal system also appears to be radiosensitive, but not to the same degree as the CNS. Skeletal abnormalities such as stunted growth, abnormal limbs, and others have been observed in the mouse fetus irradiated during the time of major organogenesis.

The incidence of prenatal death decreases when exposure occurs during major organogenesis; however, there is an increase in neonatal death (death at birth). This may be partially due to the presence of abnormalities in the fetus that are fatal at term. Table 7–4 lists some of the most common abnormalities observed in rodents and humans following in utero exposure during major organogenesis. Figures 7–8, 7–9, and 7–10 show animals with gross abnormalities resulting from in utero irradiation.

Fetal (Growth) Stage.—Irradiation during the fetal period results in fewer *obvious* abnormalities and a decreased incidence of both prenatal and neonatal deaths. Higher doses are necessary during this time to produce lethality and gross abnormalities. This is not surprising, because the cells in the fetus are more differentiated than at earlier stages of development. However, irradiation during this period of gestation may result in effects that occur later in life (e.g., cancer) or in functional disorders after birth.

TABLE 7–4.

Some Major Abnormalities Found in Mammals (Humans, Rabbits, Mice) After Fetal Irradiation*

CNS	Skeletal	Ocular	Others
Exencephaly	Stunting	Absence of eye(s)	Leukemia
Microcephaly	Abnormal limbs	Microphthalmia	Genital deformities
Mental retardation	Small head	(small eyes)	with sterility
Idiocy	Cleft palate	Strabismus	
Skull malformations	Club feet	Cataract	
Hydrocephaly	Deformed arms	Absence of lens	
Mongolism	Spina bifida		

*From Rugh R: The impact of ionizing radiation on the embryo and fetus. *Am J Roentgenol Radium Ther Nucl Med* 1963; 89:182. Used by permission.

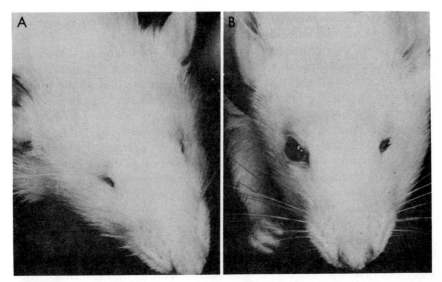

FIG 7–8.
Two rats of the same litter exposed to x-rays in utero. **A,** rat exhibiting almost total anophthalmia. **B,** rat exhibiting normal right eye but a degree of anophthalmia in the other eye. (Courtesy of Dr Roberts Rugh.)

Radiation Effects on Human Embryos

The devastating effects of radiation on the developing human embryo and fetus have been a subject of major concern for many years, and are of particular interest today with the increased use of ionizing radiation for medical purposes. This is also a very controversial subject in terms of abnormalities produced by clinical doses, especially in the diagnostic range. Many reports have appeared in the literature implicating radiation as the cause of a specific anomaly. Although it is well known that radiation does have a very dramatic effect on the fetus in terms of both lethality and the induction of congenital abnormalities, it is difficult to establish a causal relationship between radiation and a specific abnormality. Two reasons for this are as follows:

1. The incidence of spontaneous congenital abnormalities in the population is approximately 6%.
2. Radiation induces no *unique* congenital abnormalities (i.e., radiation-induced congenital abnormalities are the same as those that appear spontaneously or those caused by other factors).

These two factors make it difficult to implicate radiation as the sole cause of a specific congenital abnormality.

For obvious reasons, systematic studies of the effects of radiation on fetal development have been derived from laboratory animals, particularly mice. Although it is generally accepted that abnormalities produced in the mouse fetus by radiation also can be produced in humans, there are two factors that must be considered when extrapolating these findings to humans. One factor is time; the gestation period in mice is 20 days—in humans it is 270 days. Because the induction of specific anomalies is dependent on the period of development (gestation day) during which irradiation occurs, there will be a difference in the time these effects are induced in humans as compared to rodents.

The second important factor to consider is dose. The question is whether the human embryo is more or less sensitive than the rodent embryo. Comparative studies between mice and fruit flies (Drosophila) have shown that the more highly developed species (mouse) is more sensitive than the less developed species (fruit fly). In fact, it appears

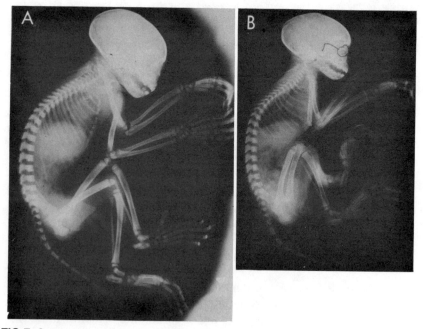

FIG 7–9.
Radiograph of 2-week-old monkey. **A,** control. **B,** animal exposed to x-rays at 13 days of gestation, indicating stunting of growth. At 13 days, the skeletal elements are differentiating. (Courtesy of Dr Roberts Rugh.)

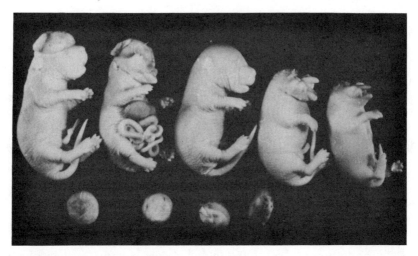

FIG 7–10.
Litter of rats exhibiting anomalies after exposure to x-rays in utero. Mother was killed at 19 days postexposure. Four fetuses were resorbed *(bottom);* the five alive exhibited, from left to right, exencephaly, exencephaly and evisceration, normalcy, and anencephaly in the last two. (Courtesy of Dr Roberts Rugh.)

that the mouse embryo is 15 times more sensitive than the fruit fly embryo. Because data on humans are rare, and dose can, at best, only be estimated in these cases, it can be assumed that the human embryo is at least as radiosensitive as the mouse embryo, if not more so.

Observations in Humans.—Radiation effects on developing human embryos have been observed in the following situations: atomic bomb survivors, accidental exposures, occupational exposures, and the diagnostic and therapeutic exposure of pregnant patients.

Congenital defects attributed to radiation in utero were described as early as 1930 by Murphy and Goldstein in a report of microcephaly related to in utero exposure. A subsequent study of the children of 106 women who received irradiation for therapeutic purposes reported that 28 of 75 of their children had radiation-induced malformations. These children exhibited both CNS and skeletal defects, including microcephalic idiocy, hydrocephaly, mental retardation without gross abnormalities, mongolism, spina bifida, double clubfoot, limb deformities, and blindness and other eye deformities. In all these cases irradiation occurred during the first trimester. However, three children irradiated after the first trimester exhibited microcephaly.

Studies of children irradiated in utero at Hiroshima show that among the offspring of eleven women who received high doses of radiation,* seven were microcephalics and mentally retarded, whereas children whose mothers were at a greater distance from the hypocenter and therefore were exposed to a lower dose did not exhibit an increased incidence of microcephaly. Of 30 children irradiated in utero at Nagasaki, there were seven fetal deaths, six neonatal deaths, and four mentally retarded children among the survivors.

In a study of the children of women irradiated with therapeutic doses during different stages of pregnancy, Dekaban draws the following conclusions:

1. Over 2.5 Gy delivered to human embryos before 2 to 3 weeks of gestation may result in a large number of prenatal deaths but produces very few severe abnormalities in those children carried to term.
2. Irradiation of the human fetus between 4 and 11 weeks of gestation may lead to severe abnormalities of many organs, particularly the CNS and skeletal systems.
3. Irradiation during the 11th to 16th weeks frequently produces mental retardation and microcephaly.
4. Although the fetus is more radioresistant in terms of lethality and abnormalities after the 20th gestational week, irradiation during this time may result in functional defects.

Follow-up of Children Irradiated In Utero at Hiroshima and Nagasaki.—More than 1,600 children irradiated in utero at Nagasaki and Hiroshima were carefully studied as they grew to maturity, providing dramatic data on the effects of irradiation at various stages of human gestation. Two major abnormalities have been observed in these surviving children: microcephaly and mental retardation.

Although accurate dose estimates are impossible, and estimated doses are problematic (in fact, the dose estimates are undergoing another revision), it is clear that doses as low as 0.09 Gy (9 rad) caused a detectable increase in the number of microcephalic individuals, regardless of the gestational age at exposure. This is particularly important as it is generally believed that microcephaly is the most common sequelae of in utero exposure after the first trimester. Table 7–5 gives the incidence of microcephaly as a function of dose for Hiroshima victims. A clear dose-response relationship was found with a clear increase observed after doses as low as 0.1 to 0.19 Gy (10 to 19 rad).

*Although doses are difficult to estimate, these women showed clinical signs of exposure to high doses.

TABLE 7–5.

Microcephaly in A-Bomb Survivors Exposed In
Utero at Hiroshima During 6 to 11 Weeks
Gestation*

Air Dose (Kerma) in Gy	Incidence	
	Percent	Number
0	4	31/764
0.01–0.09	11	2/19
0.10–0.19	17	4/24
0.20–0.29	30	3/10
0.30–0.49	40	4/10
0.50–0.99	70	7/10
1.0	100	7/7

*No excess incidence of microcephaly with exposure below
1.5 Gy in Nagasaki. Data from Committee on the Biological
Effect of Ionizing Radiations (BEIR III): The Effects on
Populations of Exposure to Low Levels of Ionizing Radia-
tion. Washington DC, National Academy of Sciences, 1980;
doses subject to review. From Hall EJ: *Radiobiology for
Radiobiologists*. Philadelphia, JB Lippincott, 1988, p 455.
Used by permission.

The incidence of mental retardation has also been reevaluated by
the committee on the Biological Effect of Ionizing Radiations (BEIR III)
committee. It was found that 30 of 1,600 children irradiated in utero
are now severely retarded, a percentage well above the normal expected
rate. The highest IQ recorded in these children was 68. Mental retardation results from exposure between the 8th and 15th week of gestation, with no increase observed if exposure occurs before 8 weeks.
The increased incidence of mental retardation following exposure between 8 and 15 weeks of gestation is consistent with the rapid proliferation of cells in the brain known to occur during this time. These
data plus the increased incidence of small head circumference indicates
that cells have been killed and subsequently depleted from the brain.

CONCLUSIONS

In general it can be stated that the embryo and fetus are more
sensitive to the effects of ionizing radiation than is the organism at any
other period of life. In addition, there are variations in the radiation
sensitivity during embryonic life. The first trimester, particularly the
first 6 weeks of development, appears to be the most radiosensitive in
terms of both lethality and induction of congenital abnormalities in
humans. The fetus becomes more resistant as development progresses

through the second and third trimesters, with higher doses necessary to produce damage.

Doses of 0.05 to 0.15 Gy that have been observed both to be fatal and to produce CNS abnormalities in mouse embryos during pre-implantation also may be damaging to human embryos during the first 2 weeks of development. However, because pregnancy in the human is generally not verified or even suspected at this early stage, and because the embryo may be resorbed by the body or aborted resulting in minimal, if any, indications of pregnancy, the implications to humans of these findings in mice are difficult to accurately assess.

The most radiosensitive time in the development of the human fetus for the induction of abnormalities is from the 2nd through the 6th week, particularly the 23rd through the 37th day of gestation. If irradiation occurs in this time interval, the greatest variety of abnormalities will be observed. As in the mouse, most radiation-induced congenital abnormalities in the human are related to the CNS. The most common abnormalities that have been observed in humans are microcephaly, mental retardation, sense organ damage, and stunted growth. The 3rd through the 20th week of human gestation appears to be the most sensitive period for skeletal changes.

The sensitivity of the fetus during the first trimester is attributable to the large number of stem cells present during the early stages of development. The majority of abnormalities appear in the CNS and related sense organs due to the abundance and diffuseness of formative cells throughout the fetus and the exquisite radiosensitivity of these stem cells.

Fetuses in the second and third trimesters are more radioresistant than those in the first. Irradiation during the last two trimesters results in a lower incidence of abnormalities than irradiation during the first trimester. However, these latter stages of development may result in more subtle abnormalities and functional disorders (e.g., sterility) and late changes such as malignancies, particularly leukemia. In addition, children irradiated in utero with therapeutic doses during the last trimester may exhibit signs and symptoms of the bone marrow syndrome at birth.

The implications of fetal exposure from the medical uses of ionizing radiation will be discussed in following chapters.

Table 7–6 summarizes all of the data on radiation effects on the embryo and fetus. It is clear that the abnormalities and risks observed are different depending on the stage of gestation in which exposure occurred. Death is the most prevalent effect of irradiation during the first trimester, while the major risk from low doses after this time is

TABLE 7–6.
Summary of Radiation Effects on the Embryo and Fetus*

Stage of Gestation	Growth Retardation	Death	Congenital Malformations	
			General	Microcephaly and Mental Retardation in Humans
Preimplantation	None	Embryonic death and resorption	None	None
Organogenesis	Temporary	Neonatal death	High risk	Very high risk
Fetal	Permanent	LD_{50} approaches that for adult	Lower risk	High risk

*From Hall EJ: *Radiobiology for the Radiobiologist.* Philadelphia, JB Lippincott Co, 1988.

CNS abnormalities. The BEIR III committee found that these changes occurred after doses as low as 0.1 Gy (10 rad) if exposure occurred during a sensitive stage of gestation.

REFERENCES

1. Bacq ZM: *Fundamentals of Radiobiology,* ed 2. New York, Pergamon Press, 1961.
2. Behrens CS, et al: *Atomic Medicine,* ed 5. Baltimore, Williams & Wilkins, 1969.
3. Bond VP, et al: *Mammalian Radiation Lethality: A Disturbance of Cellular Kinetics.* New York, Academic Press, 1965.
4. Bonte RJ: Chernobyl retrospective. *Sem Nucl Med* 1988; 18:16–24.
5. Champlin R: The role of bone marrow transplantation for nuclear accidents: Implication of the Chernobyl disaster. *Sem Hematol* 1987; 24:1–4.
6. Committee on the Biological Effects of Ionizing Radiation (BEIR III). The Effects on Populations of Exposure to Low Levels of Ionizing Radiation. Washington DC, National Academy of Sciences, 1980.
7. Dekaban AS: Abnormalities in children exposed to x-radiation during various stages of gestation: Tentative timetable of radiation injury to the human fetus. *J Nucl Med* 1968; 9:471.
8. Hempelmann LH, et al: Acute radiation syndrome: Study of 9 cases and review of problem. *Ann Intern Med* 1952; 36:279.
9. Linnemann RE: Soviet medical response to the Chernobyl nuclear accident. *JAMA* 1987; 258:637–643.
10. Lushbaugh CC: Reflections on some recent progress in human radiobiology, in Augestein LG (ed): *Advances in Radiation Biology.* New York, Academic Press, 1969, pp 277–314.
11. Miller RW, Mulvihill JJ: Small head size after atomic irradiation, in Sever JL, Brent RL (ed): *Teratogen Update, Environmentally Induced Birth Defect Risks.* New York, Alan R Liss, 1986, pp 141–143.

12. Murphy DP: *Congenital Malformations.* Philadelphia, JB Lippincott, 1947.
13. Murphy DP, Goldstein L: Micromelia in a child irradiated in utero. *Surg Gynecol Obstet* 1930; 50:79.
14. Otake M, Schull WJ: In utero exposure to A-bomb radiation and mental retardation: A reassessment. *Br J Radiol* 1984; 57:409–414.
15. Plummer C: Anomalies occurring in children exposed in utero to the atomic bomb at Hiroshima. *Pediatrics* 1952; 10:687.
16. Rugh R: *From Conception to Birth; The Drama of Life's Beginnings.* New York, Harper & Row, 1971.
17. Rugh R: The impact of ionizing radiation on the embryo and fetus. *Am J Roentgenol Radium Ther Nucl Med* 1963; 89:182.
18. Rugh R: Ionizing radiations: Their possible relation to the etiology of some congenital anomalies in human disorders. *Milit Med* 1959; 124:401.
19. Rugh R: Low levels of x-irradiation and the early mammalian embryo. *Am J Roentgenol Radium Ther Nucl Med* 1962; 87:559.
20. Rugh R: Why radiobiology? *Radiology* 1964; 82:917.
21. Rugh R: X-ray induced teratogenesis in the mouse and its possible significance to man. *Radiology* 1971; 99:433.
22. Rugh R, Grupp E: Ionizing radiations and congenital anomalies in vertebrate embryos. *Acta Embryol Exp* 1959; 2:257.
23. Rugh R, Wohlfromm M: Age of mother and previous breeding history and the incidence of x-ray induced congenital anomalies. *Radiat Res* 1963; 19:261.
24. Russell LB, Montgomery CS: Radiation sensitivity differences with cell-division cycles during mouse cleavage. *Int J Radiat Biol* 1966; 10:151.
25. Russell LB, Russell WL: An analysis of the changing radiation response of the developing mouse embryo. *J Cell Physiol* 1954; 43(suppl 1):103.
26. Thoma GE Jr, Wald N: Acute radiation syndrome in man, in *Fundamentals of Radiological Health*, Training Manual of the National Center for Radiological Health, U.S. Department of Health, Education and Welfare, DHEW Training Publication No 3n.
27. Wald N, et al: Hematologic manifestations of radiation exposure in man, *Prog Hematol* 1962; 3:1.
28. Wilson R: A visit to Chernobyl. *Science* 1987; 236:1636–1640.
29. Yamazaki JN, et al: Outcome of pregnancy in women exposed to the atomic bomb in Nagasaki. *J Dis Child* 1954; 87:448.

Chapter 8 _____

Late Effects of Radiation

_____

The previous chapter discussed the immediately lethal effects produced in the human adult and fetus by an acute high dose of radiation (greater than 1 Gy). Although knowledge of these lethal effects is necessary, incidents resulting in doses sufficiently high to cause death are relatively few. Of equal, if not more, importance are the effects observed years later in individuals who survive these acute doses.

Because the damage induced by radiation is insidious and is often manifested after long periods of time, the effects to be discussed in this chapter are such "late effects" of radiation. Unlike the immediate effects of an acute high dose, late effects remain dormant for many years and, in fact, may not be seen in the individual who was irradiated, but in succeeding generations. Thus, late effects fall into two categories. Those occurring in an exposed individual, somatic effects, and those observed in succeeding generations, genetic effects. Whereas the genetic effects of radiation so far have had to be determined from animal studies, there are sufficient human data available to allow at least some general assessment of the risk associated with the induction of cancer as a result of exposure to radiation.

Late effects do not occur only in those individuals who survive acute high dose exposures, but more importantly may be induced by single low doses and chronic low doses of radiation (low doses given over a long period of time), such as those received by patients receiving diagnostic radiology and nuclear medicine procedures or by occupationally exposed persons. In this group of individuals these effects are even more insidious, because there are no acute effects that mark these individuals for future study.

WHAT ARE "LATE EFFECTS"?

Late effects differ from the types of injury discussed previously in a number of important ways. First, unlike the types of damage produced in cells, tissues, and organs described in previous chapters, all of which was assumed to be due to cell killing, late effects arise in those cells which *survive* the initial exposure but nonetheless retain some memory of this exposure. "Late effects" such as carcinogenesis are *all or nothing events that do not exhibit a dose threshold*. Consequently, any dose, *no matter how small*, carries a probability, albeit small, of inducing the effect. Increasing the dose will increase the *probability* that this effect will occur, but it will not increase the severity of a particular late effect. Such *non-threshold effects* are termed *stochastic (i.e., random) events*. All of the changes in tissues and organs described previously exhibited a dose threshold, i.e., a dose below which the damage was not observed, but above this dose threshold the *severity* of the damage increased. Such threshold effects are termed *non-stochastic effects.*

SOMATIC EFFECTS

Carcinogenesis

The single most important late somatic effect induced by radiation is carcinogenesis, particularly after low doses such as those received by occupationally exposed personnel or by patients undergoing diagnostic tests using radiation.

Radiation has long been known to be a carcinogen (a cancer-inducing agent). The first reported case of radiation-induced carcinoma was in 1902 on the hand of a radiology technician. Within 15 years of the discovery of x-rays, 100 cases of skin cancer caused by radiation were reported in occupationally exposed personnel, both radiologists and technicians. Many famous pioneer workers and scientists in this field are thought to have died from radiation-induced cancer. Marie Curie and her daughter Irene both are thought to have died of leukemia as a result of their exposure to radiation during their experiments. Radiation then has a long history of a relationship to an increased incidence of many different types of malignancies in humans.

What Is the Risk?

The single most important question asked by individuals exposed to nonlethal doses of radiation is, "What are my chances (what is the risk) of developing cancer?" This is not an easy question to answer, particularly because the time between irradiation and the appearance of cancer is very long indeed and differs for different types of cancers. For example, the increased incidence of leukemia after irradiation of a population appears to peak between 7 and 12 years, but essentially returns to control incidence by 20 years after exposure. Latent periods for the induction of different types of solid tumors after radiation therapy vary between 20 and 30 years. These are at best estimates, and it is generally assumed that the mean latent time for the appearance of all radiation-induced cancers is about 25 years, although leukemia clearly appears sooner.

It is also critical to know whether the individual continues to be at risk throughout his life or, if after a period of time, his risk of developing cancer returns to that in the normal population. The risk of developing some cancers after irradiation seems to be a discrete event in which the risk rises for a given period of time and then returns to the natural incidence of the disease, e.g., leukemia, as discussed above. For these cancers there is an *absolute* risk of developing the disease.

However, for some other types of radiation-induced cancer the individual may be at risk throughout his life. For these types of tumors the risk of developing the disease is *relative*, and is increased by a constant factor for all ages. To obtain these data one must follow an exposed population until all of its members have died. This has not been done to date; therefore, it is not possible to distinguish whether there is an absolute or relative risk associated with most radiation-induced cancers.

How Is Risk Estimated After Low Doses?

A critical question with a major health impact is what is the risk of increasing the cancer incidence after low dose exposures such as those received by occupationally exposed persons or by persons exposed to diagnostic procedures using radiation. Currently, the best we can do is to estimate this risk after low doses by extrapolating from high-dose data, based on appropriate models. Two such models have been proposed: the linear and the linear-quadratic.

The linear model assumes that the risk per rad is the same at high and low doses, i.e., the incidence of cancer would follow a straight line over the whole dose range (Fig 8–1). The linear quadratic model assumes that there is a smaller risk per rad at low doses, and when plotted the dose incidence curve would be concave upward (see Fig 8–1). Although this discussion might seem analogous to asking the proverbial question of how many angels can dance on the head of a pin, in fact this is a critical issue for estimating cancer risks in the occupationally exposed population. Both models will fit high-dose data reasonably well (see Fig 8–1). However, a linear extrapolation of the risk from the high-dose data would overestimate the real risk at low doses and dose rates, whereas the linear quadratic model would underestimate the risks. Neither of these models can be rejected based on experimental data, although the linear quadratic model holds the most appeal for radiobiologists because so many other cell and tissue effects follow this type of curve.

Methods of Studying Radiation-Induced Malignancies

Radiation has been implicated as an etiologic (causative) factor for cancer primarily through laboratory animal studies and statistical studies of human populations exposed to radiation. For this reason we need not rely solely on the animal data to obtain estimates of risk for the

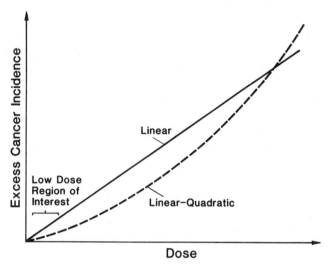

FIG 8–1.
Schematic of the linear and linear-quadratic models used to extrapolate the incidence of cancer from high-dose data to low doses. It is clear from the figure that both models fit high-dose data well, but that at low doses the estimated incidence would be dependent on the model.

carcinogenic effects of radiation, for there are sufficient numbers of incidences in which people have been exposed to radiation such that risk estimates can be based on the experience in humans. Incidence rates for cancer induced by radiation are determined by comparing the expected incidence of cancer in the control group (the general population) to the incidence in the experimental group (the irradiated population) and calculating risk factors for the irradiated population. This risk is expressed as a rate—the number of excess cancers in a defined number of individuals per unit time per unit dose. Generally, the excess risk of developing cancer after irradiation is defined as:

Number of cancer cases per 1 million (10^6) exposed people per year per rem.*

However, a number of problems arise from the statistical nature of these studies, termed epidemiologic studies (studies of disease incidence in human populations).

*A rem is a unit of dose equivalent used in radiation protection. It is defined as the dose in rads × quality factor (QF) × modifying factors (MF). QF allows for the different biologic effects of different types of radiation and is similar to RBE; MF applies primarily to internally deposited radionuclides and accounts for variations in the mode and site of deposition.

First, the observed incidence of the disease in the experimental (in this case, irradiated) population is compared with the expected incidence in the general population. This comparison is certainly valid when the experimental population consists of nondiseased individuals (e.g., in studies on radiologists). However, an experimental population consisting of diseased individuals (e.g., individuals treated with radiation for ankylosing spondylitis) may not constitute a valid comparison.

Second, the actual number of persons with cancer in the general population appears to be large but, when compared with the total number of persons in the general population, it constitutes only a small segment. Because of these small numbers, an increase in the number of cancer cases, although appearing to be large, may not be statistically significant.

Third, studies of this type cannot, by their nature, exclude other factors that may play a part in causing the observed increase in a specific disease.

Last, and very importantly, the dosimetry in most cases can, at best, only be estimated.

The first section of this chapter presents the evidence, both from animal and human studies, implicating radiation as an etiologic factor in cancer. Because the incidence of radiation-induced malignancies in humans can be documented, this section will briefly discuss these experiences.

Animal Data

Many studies using experimental animals show an increased incidence of a wide variety of malignancies after irradiation. Figure 8–2 shows one of the often-cited studies on the incidence of leukemia following a wide range of radiation doses to the total bodies of mice. This curve is characteristic of all animal carcinogenesis data: an increased incidence over a low-dose range followed by a decreased incidence after high doses, representing two different processes. After low doses the cells are not killed, but survive only to undergo malignant transformation later on. After high doses, the cells do not get an opportunity to express any malignant change because they are killed by the radiation. Although such a complete data set (i.e., over a wide dose range) is not available for humans, the fact that all experimental animal data exhibit the same shape of curve suggests that one might expect the same phenomenon to occur in humans.

Human Data

The following are sources of data on the incidence of radiation-induced cancer in humans:

1. Occupational exposure.
2. Atomic bomb survivors.
3. Medical exposure.
4. Fallout accidents in the Pacific Testing Grounds.

Malignancies in which radiation has been implicated as a cause are leukemia, skin carcinoma, osteosarcoma (cancer of the bone), and lung, thyroid, and breast cancers.

Leukemia.—The role of radiation as a cause of leukemia was first noted in 1911 in a report of 11 cases in which radiation was implicated as being leukemogenic (leukemia causing) in occupationally exposed individuals. Since that time, radiation has been definitely linked to leukemia from studies of adult populations such as atomic bomb survivors and patients treated with radiation for ankylosing spondylitis. For this reason, of all the cancers suggested to be related to radiation exposure, the best established risk estimate is that for leukemia.

Interestingly, radiation increases the incidence of only specific types of leukemia; only acute and chronic myeloid leukemia have been found to be increased in irradiated adults, whereas an increase in acute lym-

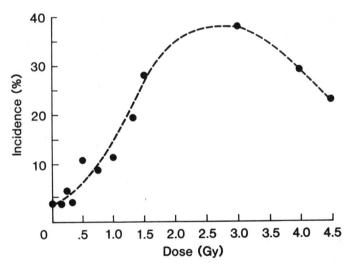

FIG 8–2.
Incidence of leukemia in male mice exposed to total-body x-irradiation. Leukemia incidence decreases after doses >3 Gy, which is due to increasing lethality after this and higher doses. (From Upton AC: The dose-response relation in radiation-induced cancer. *Cancer Res* 1961; 21:717–729. Used by permission.)

phatic leukemia is responsible for the increased incidence in exposed children. The incidence of chronic lymphocytic leukemia does not appear to be influenced by radiation exposure.

Survivors of Hiroshima and Nagasaki.—Studies of the atomic bomb survivors in both Hiroshima and Nagasaki show a statistically significant increase in leukemia incidence in the exposed population, as compared with the nonexposed population. In the period from 1950 to 1956, 117 new cases of leukemia were reported in the Japanese survivors; approximately 64 of these can be attributed to radiation exposure. In Hiroshima there was an observed frequency of 61 leukemia deaths compared with an expected incidence of 12—a fivefold increase. In Nagasaki there were 20 deaths attributable to leukemia compared with an expected rate of 7—a threefold increase.

An increased leukemia incidence also has been observed in the population exposed to low doses (0.2 to 0.5 Gy) at Hiroshima but not at Nagasaki. This difference in leukemia incidence in the two populations may be due to the different types of radiation to which they were exposed; at Nagasaki, approximately 90% of the dose was due to x-rays, while at Hiroshima about half the dose was from x-rays and half from neutrons.*

Persons Treated for Ankylosing Spondylitis.—Patients with ankylosing spondylitis treated with radiation in Great Britain comprise the second major population implicating radiation as being leukemogenic. From 1935 to 1944, approximately 15,000 patients were treated with both acute and fractionated doses ranging from 1 to 20 Gy, often to the spine and pelvis. Two-year follow-up of the patients revealed seven cases of leukemia compared with an expected incidence in the general population of one. An increase in leukemia incidence of over 100% was observed among patients who received doses greater than 20 Gy. Although the dosimetry in this situation was good, these studies are still far from ideal. First, the population observed was initially ill and consisted primarily of males,[†] which could cause an overestimate of risk when compared with the whole population. Secondly, an appropriate control group—a group of persons with the same disease but not treated with radiation—does not exist. In spite of these two limitations, these data comprise one of the largest bodies of data on leukemia

---

*Neutrons have a higher RBE than x-rays, making them biologically more damaging than x-rays.
[†]Males appear to be more susceptible than females.

in humans after radiation exposure and does show an increase, albeit small, in the incidence of this type of cancer.

Radiologists.—Another group often cited as having radiation as a causal factor in leukemia are the early radiologists. A study of 425 radiologists in the United States who died between 1948 and 1961 revealed an incidence of 12 cases of leukemia compared with an expected incidence in the general population of 4 cases; all were of the types known to be increased by radiation. However, a study of British radiologists entering practice both before and after 1921 revealed no excess in leukemia incidence, thereby refuting the findings in American radiologists and shedding doubt on the conclusion of that study. It is now accepted that the incidence of leukemia in radiologists is not higher than in other medical specialties nor in the general population.

Skin Carcinoma.—Several radiation reactions were reported on the hands of early radiologists and technicians soon after Röntgen's discovery, with the first case of skin cancer reported in 1902 on the hand of a technician. Because their x-ray machines were crude, radiologists placed their hands in the beam to check the efficiency, resulting in high exposure to the hands, with a large number of individuals developing skin carcinoma years later. In fact, 100 cases of skin cancer had been reported in radiologists and technicians 15 years after the discovery of x-rays. Another source of information regarding radiation-induced skin cancer is individuals treated with radiation for acne and ringworm; many developed skin cancer years later.

Although skin carcinoma caused by radiation cannot be differentiated from skin cancer caused by other agents, enough evidence exists to implicate radiation as a definite cause. What must be kept in mind concerning both these groups is that they were exposed to unfiltered low-kV x-rays that produce extremely high doses in the superficial layers of the skin. Because of these incidents in pioneer workers, which resulted in safety precautions on x-ray units and a reduction in maximum permissible doses (MPD), radiation-induced skin cancer has disappeared in occupationally exposed persons.

Osteosarcoma (Bone Cancer).—The story of the watch dial painters in the early part of this century (1915 to 1930), who pointed their brushes with their lips, is well known. Radium, used to paint the clock faces, was ingested by these workers in this manner and, because radium is a bone-seeker, accumulated in the skeleton. Although exposure to the radioactive material was brief, the ingested radium was not ex-

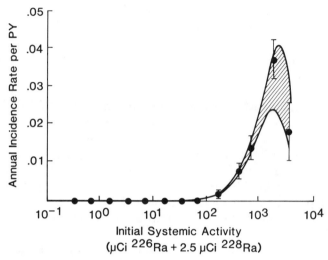

FIG 8–3.
Semilogarithmic plot of the incidence of bone sarcoma in the radium dial painters as a function of dose. The shaded band indicates ± one standard deviation of the fit to the data. (From Rowland R, Stehney AF, Lucas HF: Dose-response relationships for radium-induced bone sarcomas. *Health Phys* 1983; 44:15–31. Used by permission.)

creted, resulting in a continuous exposure to the bone. As a result, approximately 40 of a total of several hundred persons developed osteosarcoma—a much greater than expected incidence. Figure 8–3 shows the dose response data from the studies on these workers, indicating that the linear-quadratic model best fits these data (see Fig 8–1).

Lung Carcinoma.—Pitchblende miners in Germany more than 500 years ago were known to have a high incidence of a fatal disease referred to as "mountain sickness." In 1924, investigation of this disease revealed it to be carcinoma of the lung. The cause of the disease was occupational and partially attributable to the fact that the air in the pitchblende mines was rich in radon.

An increased incidence of lung cancer was also reported among uranium miners in the western United States. A study of miners from 1950 to 1967 revealed 62 cases of lung cancer, six times the expected number. This number was also increased over the number of lung cancers reported in other types of miners. These tumors are believed to be caused by the inhalation and subsequent deposition in the lungs of dust containing radioactive material.

Thyroid Carcinoma.—The practice of irradiating the thymus in infants to reduce "thymic enlargement" gained popularity in the early decades of this century and declined after the 1930s. Doses to these infants ranged from 1.2 to 60 Gy, and resulted in a hundredfold increase in the incidence of thyroid cancer in this group. Although there is not sufficient data on children with the same disease who were not irradiated to allow a valid comparison of the effects induced by radiation and those caused by the disease itself, all studies of this group reveal a significantly higher incidence of thyroid cancer in the irradiated than in the nonirradiated population.

Another source of information concerning thyroid cancer attributable to radiation is the children of the Marshall Islanders who were accidentally exposed to fallout radiation from a nuclear test device when a sudden wind shift occurred at the time of testing. In later years these irradiated children revealed an increased incidence of all types of thyroid disease, including benign and malignant tumors. Follow-up studies of the survivors at Hiroshima and Nagasaki also have shown an increased incidence of thyroid cancer in those individuals who were children at the time of the bombing. Although doses are difficult to determine in the above situations, estimates reveal that a dose of 1.0 Gy or less had been received by some individuals who later developed thyroid cancer. The latent period for this radiation-induced cancer appears to be 10 to 20 years.

Breast Cancer.—A study of three groups of irradiated women has shown conclusively that radiation increases the incidence of breast cancer. These groups are:

1. Female survivors of the atomic bomb attacks in Hiroshima and Nagasaki.
2. Canadian women with tuberculosis who were subjected to multiple fluoroscopies.
3. Women treated for benign breast diseases such as postpartum mastitis.

Because of the large sample size and reasonable estimates of the dosimetry and doses received, the Canadian study constitutes strong evidence that radiation can cause breast cancer.

Figure 8–4 shows the data from the Canadian study. These data can be reasonably fitted by a straight line, suggesting that the incidence of at least this one type of cancer would be *linearly* related to dose.

Other Malignancies.—Although the above cancers are those most often attributed to radiation, radiation has been implicated as an etiologic factor for other cancers, such as salivary gland cancer and some sarcomas.

In Utero Exposure and Cancer.—Radiation exposure during fetal life had long been suggested as increasing the incidence of cancer. This suggestion was based on two studies, one in England, the much quoted study of Stewart and co-workers, and a second in the United States, another often-cited study by MacMahon. On closer scrutiny of these studies, their data, and conclusions, a number of problems have become apparent. It is now well accepted that neither of these studies clearly demonstrates a causal relationship between in utero exposure and cancer in the child.

This conclusion is supported by two independent data sets. First, in the Stewart study, the siblings of those children exposed in utero who later died of cancer had a cancer incidence twice that of the siblings of the control group, i.e., children not irradiated in utero. Secondly, those Japanese children irradiated in utero during the bombing of Nagasaki and Hiroshima have shown no increase in the incidence of childhood cancers. However, because of the exquisite sensitivity of the developing embryo and fetus, and to be conservative and safe, it is suggested that a value of 1.5 to 2 be used to estimate the increased risk

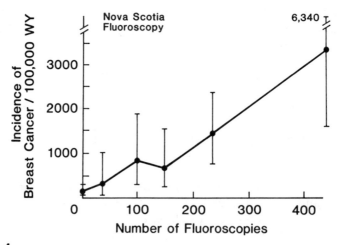

FIG 8–4.
Incidence of breast cancer as a function of the number of fluoroscopies, from the Canadian study showing a linear relationship between cancer induction and radiation dose for at least this one type of cancer. (From Boice JD, Land CE, Shore RE, et al: Risk of breast cancer following low dose exposure. *Radiology* 1979; 131:589–597. Used by permission.)

of inducing malignancy after fetal irradiation than after irradiation of an adult.

How Does Radiation Induce Cancer?

Although radiation has been shown to increase the incidence of cancer, the reasons for its doing so remain speculative. Structural changes in chromosomes resulting in mutations are a known effect of radiation. Although it is certainly possible that a mutated cell may be the responsible agent, the probability of a mutation in one or a few cells resulting in a malignancy is small.

One likely and current hypothesis is that radiation, via the translocation of genetic material, allows oncogenes normally unexpressed to be expressed, ultimately causing cancer. (Oncogenes are genes whose expression is speculatively linked to the conversion of normal cells to cancer cells.) This is one reasonable hypothesis, particularly since chromosome translocations have been found in some naturally occurring human tumors. However, such circumstantial evidence does not prove cause and effect, nor does it eliminate the expressed oncogene hypothesis.

It will more likely be found that a combination of many factors play a role in inducing cancer. In addition, other environmental and health factors that increase the risk of cancer have been identified; more of these undoubtedly will be identified in the future. The present evidence implies that radiation is one of many insults, not the sole factor, in the etiology of cancer, particularly in view of current low exposures to all individuals. The mechanism by which radiation induces cancer remains elusive and controversial.

Conclusions

The fact that radiation causes cancer cannot be disputed. The major controversy concerns dose information; in most instances, only estimates are available. Doses as low as 0.25 Gy have been implicated as causing malignancies in adults, whereas in utero exposure doses causing malignancies are lower. The fact that infants and children are generally more radiosensitive may imply that lower doses will cause more cancer in the young than in adults; an even lower dose may cause cancer in the radiosensitive fetus.

Latent periods vary with the type of cancer studied and range from 5 to 30 years. Whether radiation-induced cancers follow a linear or linear-quadratic function with dose is unknown in most cases, and will probably differ for different malignancies. For example, the breast cancer data indicate that the incidence of this disease does follow a linear

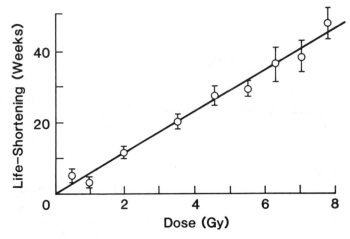

FIG 8–5.
Life-span shortening in mice as a function of radiation dose. (From Rotblat J, Lindop P: Long-term effects of a single whole body exposure of mice to ionizing radiation, II. Causes of death. *Proc R Soc London [Biol]* 1961; 154:332. Used by permission.)

relationship with dose, whereas a linear relationship would not fit the radium dial painter bone sarcoma data well. Also, the incidence of some cancers will follow an absolute risk model, e.g., leukemia, which peaks between 7 and 12 years after exposure but returns to normal by 20 years. However, for other types of cancer, exposed individuals may well be at risk all their lives.

Today, in general, the incidence of radiation-induced cancer appears to be decreasing, a trend that may be attributed to two factors:

1. The knowledge of these dangerous effects, which has led to strict regulations regarding usage and a lowering of MPDs to occupationally exposed personnel and the general population.
2. The cessation of the misuse of radiation as a panacea for treating illnesses of all types.

NONSPECIFIC LIFE SHORTENING

Studies in small animals have shown that animals chronically exposed to low doses of radiation die younger than animals never exposed to radiation (Fig 8–5). Examination of these animals at death revealed a decrease in the numbers of parenchymal cells and blood vessels and an increase in connective tissue in organs—indications of an aging process. This phenomenon is often referred to as radiation-induced aging because it appears to be an acceleration of the aging process.

However, larger scale studies on experimental animals conducted in the United States have shown that although radiation does shorten the normal life span, these earlier deaths are due to specific, not general, causes. After moderate doses, cancer induction accounts for the reduced life span. Higher doses do, indeed, cause an "aging" process, i.e., atrophy of organs and degenerative changes, most likely due to cell killing and subsequent cell loss (see Chapters 4 and 6).

Thus, radiation does not cause a nonspecific accelerated aging and a subsequent shortening of life. Rather, the earlier deaths are due to the induction of cancer.

GENETIC EFFECTS

Although somatic late effects are unfortunate for the afflicted individuals, of equal if not greater consequence is the impact of radiation exposure on future generations. In fact, for many years the hazards and risks to future generations were believed to be of much greater consequence than those to the individual; this belief is being questioned today.

Genetics and the function of DNA as the storehouse of all genetic information were discussed in Chapter 1. It was also pointed out that genes and the sequence of bases on the DNA chain are stable, i.e., during both mitosis and meiosis, DNA makes a duplicate of itself, which is transmitted to the daughter cells thus maintaining the integrity of genetic information in the cell. This process is extremely important in germ cells, which transmit the information to future generations.

Occasionally, for some unknown reason, genes and DNA spontaneously change, altering either the structure or the amount of DNA in the cell. These naturally occurring changes, termed *spontaneous mutations*, are permanent and heritable, i.e., they may be passed from cell to cell and possibly from generation to generation.

Generally thought to be detrimental, the effect of mutations on the individual depend on the gene in which the change has occurred. Some genes are vital to life, therefore a mutation in these genes is severely detrimental, possibly resulting in the death of the individual before adulthood. Mutations in less vital genes are of less consequence to the life of the individual. Examples of spontaneous mutations in the human population are mongoloids and hydrocephalics.

A certain number of spontaneous mutations arise in each generation; this is termed the *mutation frequency*. The frequency of spontaneous mutations in a generation can be altered by a number of factors including viruses, chemicals, and radiation. These agents, termed *mutagens*, are responsible for increasing the spontaneous mutation rate.

Radiation certainly can produce mutations through unrepaired structural breaks in chromosomes or through discrete changes in the order of bases on the DNA chain (Chapter 2). When these mutations occur in germ cells, the possibility exists that they may be transmitted to future generations. Chapter 7 discussed the effects of in utero irradiation on the fetus; this section will discuss the second way in which radiation affects the fetus and therefore future generations through the transmission of a radiation-induced mutation in the ovum or sperm. This category comprises the genetic effects of radiation.

Methods of Studying Radiation-Induced Mutations

The effect of radiation on mutation frequency has been studied extensively in laboratory animals, primarily in the fruit fly and mouse. As in studying other effects of radiation, it is not possible to subject humans to the controlled conditions necessary for determining these effects. In the study of genetic effects, breeding is controlled—only certain males are permitted to mate with specific females because of their characteristics. The offspring are then studied for the presence or absence of these characteristics. A second important factor in studying genetic effects is the life span of the individuals in the species. Because genetic effects are not necessarily exhibited in the first generation of offspring, many generations must be observed, necessitating a short life span. Most laboratory animals used for genetic studies fit this criterion. In addition, the laboratory animals used give birth to multiple offspring per mating, an unusual situation in humans. This larger number of offspring increases the probability of observing genetic effects.

Doubling Dose

The unit of measurement for the determination of radiation effect on mutation frequency is the *doubling dose,* defined as that dose of radiation which ultimately doubles the number of spontaneous mutations. For example, if 5% of the offspring in each generation are observed to have mutations, the doubling dose would eventually produce 10% mutations. Because radiation produces no new mutations, only an increase in the already existing number of mutations is observed.

Animal Data

The classic study of the effect of radiation on mutation frequency

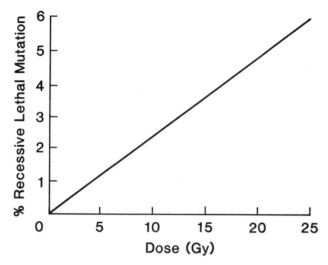

FIG 8–6.
The percentage of recessive lethal mutations in the fruit fly as a function of radiation dose. (From Hall EJ: *Radiobiology for the Radiologist.* New York, Harper & Row, 1973, p 222. Used by permission.)

was done in 1927 by Herman J. Müller in a comprehensive study of fruit flies (*Drosophilia melanogaster*). By exposing males and females to various doses of radiation, observing lethality and the change in appearance of the offspring of irradiated parents, and comparing these results with unirradiated controls, Müller drew the following conclusions pertaining to fruit flies:

1. Radiation did not produce any new or unique mutations—it simply increased the number of mutations that spontaneously arise in each generation.
2. Between doses of 0.25 and 4 Gy, the frequency of mutations was linear with dose. Equal dose increments produced an equal increase in the number of mutations.
3. Radiation-induced mutations were recessive, i.e., they may not be exhibited for many generations.*
4. The incidence of radiation-induced mutations did not exhibit a dose threshold, meaning that ultimately any dose, no matter how small, could produce a mutation (Fig 8–6).
5. The incidence of mutations was independent of dose rate. In Müller's study, a given dose produced the same incidence of mutations, whether it was given as one "shot" of radiation or

---

*For a recessive mutation to be expressed in an individual, the same mutated gene must be received from both parents, an unlikely event.

extended over a long period of time, suggesting that radiation-induced mutations are cumulative.

6. The doubling dose for humans extrapolated from the *Drosophila* data was estimated to be between 5 and 150 rem.

Although these studies provided valuable and new information on radiation-induced mutations, nonetheless it's difficult, if not impossible, to extrapolate data from such studies to humans, particularly the conclusions concerning the doubling dose. Succinctly stated by Neel: "Many of the conclusions derived from experiments with *Drosophila* (fruit fly) and mice . . . cannot be interpolated because man is neither an over-grown fruit fly nor an oversized mouse."

Prompted by the dropping of the atomic bombs on Japan, in the 1950s it became pertinent to obtain more information on the genetic effects of radiation in humans using a more appropriate model than the fruit fly, but retaining the strengths of this model, i.e., short life span, easily recognizable mutations, and the ability to screen large numbers of subjects at relatively small cost. The husband-and-wife team of Russell and Russell at Oak Ridge National Laboratory in the United States undertook such a study using a mouse strain with an easily identifiable mutation that was increased by radiation. Because they used thousands of mice, this project is often referred to as the megamouse experiment.

Neither their efforts nor the mice's were in vain, however, for the data from these studies critical to human radiation genetics were not in agreement with those data from the fruit fly experiment. The important findings from the megamouse studies were:

1. There *was* a clear dose rate effect in the mouse for radiation-induced mutations; when a given dose was extended over a period of time it produced fewer mutations than the same dose given in one single shot. This finding was directly opposite to the fruit fly data, in which no dose rate effect was observed.

2. Based on these data, the doubling dose for humans was estimated to be 50 to 250 rem, significantly higher than that estimated from the fruit fly data.

These two findings alone justified the studies, for they clearly changed the then-held thinking on radiation-induced mutations in humans.

In addition, three other conclusions were drawn from these data that were critical and relevant to humans:

1. All mutations did not show the same susceptibility to induction by radiation, indicating that the doubling dose is not a constant for all types of mutations, but will vary with the mutation studied.
2. Males were found to be more sensitive than females, particularly after low doses, suggesting that the burden of genetic effects in the population is carried by males.
3. These effects can be reduced by allowing a time period to elapse between exposure and conception. By extrapolating from the mouse data, 6 months is the suggested period of time in humans that should be allowed to elapse between radiation exposure and conception to reduce the probability of genetic effects.

Human Data

Because a study of the effects of radiation on mutation rate in humans is not feasible, most information concerning these effects has been extrapolated from animal studies. As Neel suggested, and what became obvious from a comparison of the fruit fly and mouse studies, is that such an extrapolation could provide erroneous information, specifically in the doubling dose.

One situation in humans that has allowed the observation of radiation-induced genetic effects is the study of children conceived after one or both parents were exposed to radiation at Hiroshima or Nagasaki. Approximately 71,000 pregnancies were entered in a study in postwar Hiroshima and Nagasaki between 1948 and 1953; the control population was Japanese people living outside these two cities. The parents were grouped according to dose, those who received a low dose (<0.1 Gy) and those who received a high dose (>1 Gy). These data showed that there was *no statistically significant increase* in the mutations studied in the irradiated population, although there was a trend toward increased incidence of mutations in the high-dose group.

Based on these data, a general doubling dose has been estimated at 156 rem (1.56 sv).

Conclusions

It is clear that radiation can increase the incidence of mutations in an exposed population. Important points to keep in mind about radiation-induced mutations are:

1. Radiation simply increases the incidence of the same muta-

tions that occur spontaneously; it does not produce new mutations.

2. The incidence of radiation-induced mutations follows a linear relationship with dose.
3. The incidence of mutations is most likely dose-rate dependent in humans.
4. Data derived from the mouse experiments are probably not too far off from those that would be relevant to humans.
5. The doubling dose is the dose required to double the spontaneous mutation rate, and has been estimated to be in the range of 50 to 250 rem by the BEIR III committee, or 1 Gy by the 1986 United National Scientific Committee on the Effects of Atomic Radiation.

To place all of this in perspective, however, it is generally accepted that in utero irradiation has a more significant impact on the health and life of the individual than does any radiation-induced genetic change.

REFERENCES

1. Albert RW, et al: Follow-up study of patients treated by x-ray epilation for tinea capitis. *Arch Environ Health* 1968; 17:899.
2. Committee on the Biological Effects of the Ionizing Radiation (BEIR III): The Effects on Populations of Exposure to Low Levels of Ionizing Radiation. Washington DC, National Academy of Sciences, 1980.
3. Boice JD Jr, Land CE, Shore RE, et al: Risk of breast cancer following low dose exposure. *Radiology* 1979; 131:589–597.
4. Boice JD, Monson RR: X-ray exposure and breast cancer. *Am J Epidemiol* 1976; 104:349–350.
5. Bross ID, Natarajan N: Leukemia from low level radiation: Identification of susceptible children. *N Engl J Med* 1972; 287:107.
6. Conard RA, et al: Thyroid nodules as a late sequela of radioactive fallout, in a Marshall Island population exposed in 1954. *N Engl J Med* 1966; 274:1391.
7. Conard RA, et al: Thyroid neoplasia as late effect of exposure to radioactive iodine in fallout. *JAMA* 1970; 214:316.
8. Conard RA, Hicking A: Medical findings in Marshallese people exposed to fallout radiation: Results from a ten-year study. *JAMA* 1965; 192:457.
9. *Court-Brown WM, Doll R: Expectation of life and mortality from cancer among British radiologists. *Br Med J* 1958; 2(5090):181.
10. Court-Brown WM, Doll R: Mortality from cancer and other causes after radiotherapy for ankylosing spondylitis. *Br Med J* 1965; 2(5474):1327.

*Court-Brown WM is occasionally indexed as Brown WM.

11. Court-Brown WM, et al: The incidence of leukaemia after the exposure to diagnostic radiation in utero. *Br Med J* 1960; 2(5212):1599.

12. Curtis HJ: *Radiation-Induced Aging in Mice*, Third Australasian Conference on Radiobiology, University of Sydney, 1958. London: Butterworth, 1961, pp 114–22.

13. Dublin LI, Spiegelman M: Mortality of medical specialists, 1938–1942. *JAMA* 1948; 137:1519.

14. Evans RD, et al: Radiogenic tumors in the radium and mesothorium cases studied at MIT, in May CW, et al (eds): *Delayed Effects of Bone-Seeking Radionuclides*. Salt Lake City, University of Utah Press, 1969, p. 157.

15. Ford DD, et al: Fetal exposure to diagnostic x-rays and leukemia and other malignant diseases in childhood. *J Natl Cancer Inst* 1959; 22:1093.

16. Fujita S, Awa AA, Pierce DA, et al: Re-evaluation of the biological effects of radiation by the changes of estimation of dose, in *Proc Int Symp on Biological Effects of Low Level Radiation with Special Regard to Stochastic and Non-Stochastic Effects*. Vienna, IAEA, 1983.

17. Griem ML, et al: Analysis of the morbidity and mortality of children irradiated in fetal life. *Radiology* 1967; 88:347.

18. Hall EJ: *Radiobiology for the Radiologist*, ed 3. New York: Harper & Row, 1988.

19. Härting FH, Hesse W: Der Lungekrebs, die Berkrankheit in den Schneeberger Gruben. *Vrljschr Gerichtl Med* 1879; 30:296; 31:102, 313.

20. Hempelmann LH: Risk of thyroid neoplasms after irradiation in childhood: Studies of populations exposed to radiation in childhood show a dose response over a wide dose range. *Science* 1968; 160:159.

21. Ju DM: Salivary gland tumors occurring after irradiation of the head and neck area. *Am J Surg* 1968; 116:518.

22. Krall JF: Estimation of spontaneous and radiation induced mutation rates in man. *Eugenics Q* 1956; 3:201.

23. MacMahon B: Prenatal x-ray exposure and childhood cancer. *J Natl Cancer Inst* 1962; 28:1173.

24. MacMahon B, Newill VA: Birth characteristics of children dying of malignant neoplasms. *J Natl Cancer Inst* 1962; 28:231.

25. March HC: Leukemia in radiologists. *Radiology* 1944; 43:275.

26. March HC: Leukemia in radiologists in a 20-year period. *Am J Med Sci* 1950; 220:282.

27. Martland HS: Occurrence of malignancy in radioactive persons; general review of data gathered in study of radium dial painters, with special reference to occurrence of osteogenic sarcoma and interrelationship of certain blood diseases. *Am J Cancer* 1931; 15:2435.

28. McKenzie I: Breast cancer following multiple fluoroscopies. *Br J Cancer* 1965; 19:1.

29. Miller RW: Delayed radiation effects in atomic-bomb survivors; Major observations by the Atomic Bomb Casualty Commission are evaluated. *Science* 1969; 166:569.

30. Mole RH: Radiation effects in man: Current views and prospects. *Health Phys* 1971; 20:485.
31. Morgan KZ: Biological effects of ionizing radiation. Lecture, presented at "Environmental Analysis and Environmental Monitoring for Nuclear Power Generation," University of California, Berkeley, September 9–13, 1974.
32. Müller HJ: Artificial transmutation of the gene. *Science* 1927; 66:84.
33. National Academy of Sciences: *Effects on Populations of Exposure to Low Levels of Ionizing Radiations*. Report of the Advisory Commission on Biological Effects of Ionizing Radiations, Division of Medical Sciences, National Academy of Sciences/National Research Council, November 1972.
34. Neel JV: *Changing Perspectives on the Genetic Effects of Radiation*. Springfield, Ill, Charles C Thomas, 1963.
35. Neel JV: On some pitfalls in developing an adequate genetic hypothesis. *Am J Human Genet* 1955; 7(1):1.
36. Pack GT, Davis J: Radiation cancer of the skin. *Radiology* 1965; 84:436.
37. Petersen O: Radiation cancer: Report of 21 cases. *Acta Radiol (Stockh)* 1954; 42(3):221.
38. Rotblat J, Lindop P: Long-term effects of a single whole body exposure of mice to ionizing radiation. II. Causes of death. *Proc R Soc Lond [Biol]* 1961; 154:350.
39. Rowland RE, Stehney AF, Lucas HF: Dose response relationships for radium induced bone sarcomas. *Health Phys* 1983; 44:15–31.
40. Russell WL: Genetic hazards of radiation. *Proc Am Phil Soc* 1963; 107:11.
41. Russell WL: Studies in mammalian radiation genetics. *Nucleonics* 1965; 23:53.
42. Saccomanno G, et al: Lung cancer of uranium miners on the Colorado plateau. *Health Phys* 1964; 10:1195.
43. Schull WL, Otake M, Neal JV: Genetic effects of the atomic bomb: A reappraisal. *Science* 1981; 213:1220–1227.
44. Seltser R, Sartwell PE: Influence of occupational exposure to radiation on mortality of American radiologists and other medical specialists. *Am J Epidemiol* 1965; 81:2.
45. Simpson CL, Hempelmann LH: The association of tumors and roentgenray treatment of the thorax in infancy. *Cancer* 1957; 10(1):42.
46. Socolow EL, et al: Thyroid carcinoma in man after exposure to ionizing radiation; A summary of the findings in Hiroshima and Nagasaki. *N Engl J Med* 1963; 268:406.
47. Spencer WP, Stern C: Experiments to test the validity of the linear R dose mutation frequency relationship in Drosophila at low dosage. *Genetics* 1948; 33:43.
48. Sternglass EJ: Evidence for Low Level Radiation Effects on the Human Embryo and Fetus, *Proc Ninth Hannford Biology Symposium*. Atomic Energy Commission Symposium Series 17, 1969, pp 651–60.

49. Stewart A: *An Epidemiologist Takes a Look at Radiation Risks.* US Department of Health, Education and Welfare, DHEW Publication (FDA) 73-8024, January 1973.
50. Stewart A, et al: A survey of childhood malignancies. *Br Med J* 1958; 1(5086):1495.
51. Sutow WW, Conard RA: Effects of Fallout Radiation on Marshallese Children, *Proc Ninth Hannford Biology Symposium.* Atomic Energy Commission Symposium Series 17, 1969, pp. 661–74.
52. Toyooka ET, et al: Neoplasms in children treated with x-rays for thymic enlargement. II. Tumor incidence as a function of radiation factors. *J Natl Cancer Inst* 1963; 31:1357.
53. US Congress, Joint Committee on Atomic Energy, Subcommittee on Research Development in Radiation: *Radiation Exposure of Uranium Miners* (Washington DC, US Government Printing Office, 1968).
54. United National Scientific Committee on the Effects of Atomic Radiation: *Ionizing Radiation: Sources and Biological Effects.* New York, United Nations, 1982.
55. Upton AC: Radiation carcinogenesis, in *Methods in Cancer Research,* vol. 4. New York, Academic Press, 1968.
56. Wanebo CK, et al: Breast cancer after exposure to the atomic bombings of Hiroshima and Nagasaki. *N Engl J Med* 1968; 279:667.
57. Warren S: Longevity and causes of death from irradiation in physicians. *JAMA* 1956; 162(5):464.
58. Warren S: Radiation carcinogenesis. *Bull NY Acad Med* 1970; 46:131.
59. Warren S, Lombard OM: New data on the effects of ionizing radiation on radiologists. *Arch Environ Health (Chicago)* 1966; 13:415.
60. Wolff S: Radiation genetics. *Annu Rev Genet* 1967, 1:221.

Clinical Radiobiology I: Diagnostic Radiology and Nuclear Medicine

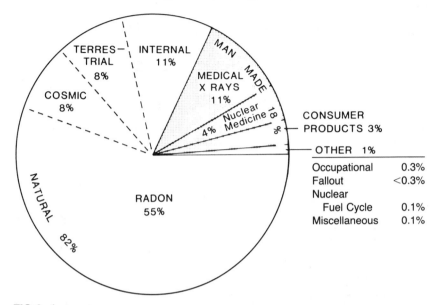

FIG 9–1.
Percent contribution of natural and man-made radiation sources to the total effective dose equivalent in the U.S. population.

The general population is exposed to ionizing radiation from two sources: natural and man-made. Natural sources of radiation include exposure from the earth's crust, outer space, building materials, and naturally occurring radioactive materials in the body. Man-made radiation sources are medical (including diagnostic radiology, nuclear medicine, and radiation therapy) and dental exposures, fallout from nuclear weapons, nuclear power industries, and occupational radiation exposures. The percentage each of these sources contributes to radiation exposure to the general population is shown in Figure 9–1. The contribution of both natural and man-made radiation sources to total body and gonadal exposure to the general population is given in Table 9–1. These data show that the greatest contribution to the exposure of the general population to radiation is from natural sources, particularly radon and its decay products. Also, it is clear that among man-made sources, medical exposures constitute the largest contributors to both total-body and gonadal radiation exposure.

Although the *number of persons* exposed to medical sources of radiation cannot be reliably estimated, the *number of medical and dental examinations* can be estimated from available data. These estimates, given in Table 9–2 for three specific years during the last 25 years (1964 to 1988), indicate that the total numbers of diagnostic med-

TABLE 9–1.

Annual Effective Dose Equivalent and GSD in the U.S. Population c. 1980 to 1982*

Source	Average Number of People Exposed (thousands)	Average Annual H_E[†] in Exposed Population (mSv)[‡]	Average Annual Collective H_E[†] (person-Sv)[§]	Contributions to GSD (mSv)[‡]	Contributions to GSD mrem
Natural sources					
Radon	230,000	2.0	460,000	.10	10
Other	230,000	1.0	230,000	.90	90
Occupational	930[¶]	2.3	2,000	.006	0.6
Nuclear fuel	—	—	136	.0005	0.05
Consumer products					
Tobacco[‖]	50,000	—	—	—	
Other	120,000	.05–0.3	12,000–29,000	.05	5
Miscellaneous environmental sources	~25,000	.006	160	.001	0.1
Medical					
Diagnostic x-rays	—[††]	—	91,000	.20–.30	20–30
Nuclear medicine	—[‡‡]	—	32,000	.02	2
Rounded totals	**230,000**	**—**	**835,000**	**1.3**	**130**

* From National Council on Radiation Protection and Measurements: *Ionizing Radiation Exposure of the Population of the United States.* Washington DC, US Government Printing Office, NCRPM Report No 93, 1987.
[†] H_E is the effective dose equivalent.
[‡] 1 mSv = 100 mrem.
[§] 1 person-Sv = 100 person-rem.
[¶] Those nominally exposed total 1.68×10^6.
[‖] Effective dose equivalent difficult to determine; dose to a segment of bronchial epithelium estimated to be 0.16 Sv/yr (16 rem/yr).
[††] Number of persons exposed is not known. Number of examinations was 180 million and H_E per examination, 500 μSv.
[‡‡] Number of persons exposed is not known. Number of examinations was 7.4 million and H_E per examination, 4,300 μSv.

TABLE 9–2.

Estimated Total Diagnostic Medical and Dental X-ray Procedures in the United States*

	Number of Examinations (in thousands)		
	1964	1970	1980
Medical	109,000	136,000	180,000
Dental	54,000	67,000	101,000
Total	163,000	203,000	281,000

*From National Council on Radiation Protection and Measurements: *Ionizing Radiation Exposure of the Population of the United States,* Washington DC, US Government Printing Office, Report No 93. Used by permission.

ical and dental x-ray procedures have nearly doubled in the last quarter century.

In view of these figures, it is interesting to reflect on an editorial that appeared in the Pall Mall Gazette (London, 1896) concerning x-rays and their use:

We are sick of the rontgen ray. . .you can see other people's bones with the naked eye, and also see through eight inches of solid wood. On the revolting indecency of this there is no need to dwell. But what we seriously put before the attention of the Government. . .that it will call for legislative restriction of the severest kind. Perhaps the best thing would be for all civilized nations to combine to burn all works on the rontgen rays, to execute all the discoverers, and to corner all the tungstate in the world and whelm it in the middle of the ocean.

It is indeed fortunate that this feeling did not gain widespread acceptance, because the use of radiation in the diagnosis of disease has become an invaluable and necessary tool in the armamentarium of every physician, regardless of specialty. At this time there is no reason to assume that the use of radiation for diagnostic purposes will decrease, even though many new developments in imaging technology, e.g., magnetic resource imaging (MRI), do not use ionizing radiation.

Although the benefits derived from diagnostic procedures cannot be disputed, the risks involved to both patients and personnel, and the principles of radiation hygiene, must be considered by all individuals administering radiation, both physicians and technologists.

All available evidence indicates that immediate medically expressed radiation damage does not occur below doses of 0.5 Gy (50 rad) in the majority of exposed individuals. Exposure to patients and personnel from diagnostic procedures falls well below this dose, into the category of low doses—the effects of which are classified as late effects and remain speculative and difficult to evaluate, as discussed in Chapter 8.

Exposure to patients is limited to one specific body area, rendering the determination of the systemic effects of these low doses even more difficult. The added factor of chronic exposure to these low doses must be considered in the case of occupationally exposed persons.

With these precautions in mind, this chapter will discuss the risks involved to patients and personnel from medical uses of radiation for diagnostic purposes, i.e., diagnostic radiology and nuclear medicine.

WHAT ARE THE RISKS?

The primary risks to the general public from the low doses of radiation received in either a medical setting or in an occupational setting are stochastic effects, particularly carcinogenic and genetic effects. Persons at risk include the individual, specifically for the risk of cancer induction; future generations, at risk for genetic effects; and the embryo and fetus, at risk for both cancer and genetic effects. Because the doses are very low, it is assumed there will be no nonstochastic effects induced (no cells will be killed by these low doses).

However, cell killing is not the only effect of radiation. Equally important is whether irradiated cell survivors retain some memory of that exposure, resulting years later in cancer or genetic effects (see Chapter 8). It must be kept in mind that there are considerable uncertainties associated with risk estimates of this type and that new information on both the genetic and carcinogenic effects of radiation constantly shapes our thinking and philosophy. Nonetheless, it is best to assume that there must be some risk involved when so many people are being irradiated.

Having said this, however, what must be kept in perspective is that radiation for diagnostic purposes is given to assist in obtaining a prompt and accurate diagnosis of a disease. What must be balanced, then, are the risks associated with the procedure vs. the potential benefit to the individual. Clearly, the prospects of causing cancer or genetic effects years later pales beside a potentially life-threatening disease that may be curable if an accurate diagnosis is speedily rendered.

TERMINOLOGY

Before proceeding with a discussion of the risks involved, it is important to have some knowledge of the terminology used to discuss the effects of low-level exposures to ionizing radiation. Because these stochastic changes affect not only the individual but also the whole population, different terms are used when discussing the risk to the individual from those used when relating these risks to the population in general. The dosimetric terms used are: (1) *dose equivalent,* (2) *effective dose equivalent,* (3) *collective dose equivalent,* and (4) *genetically significant dose.*

Dose Equivalent

Dose equivalent is defined as the absorbed dose times a quality factor. The quality factor (Q) is related to LET and allows for the fact that some kinds of radiation are more biologically harmful than others. The dose equivalent attempts to place the effects of different types of radiation on a common biologic scale. Quality factor is not the same as RBE (see Chapter 2), as there is not a common endpoint used for measuring this factor. The National Commission on Radiological Protection (NCRP) has recommended the following values for Q: for low-LET radiations, $Q = 1.0$; for neutrons, $Q = 20$; and for α-

particles, $Q = 20$. If the absorbed dose is expressed in rads, the dose equivalent is expressed in rem, if the absorbed dose is expressed in Gy, the dose equivalent is expressed in Sv.*

Effective Dose Equivalent

Effective dose equivalent (H_E) is a concept introduced by the NCRP and is an attempt to equate the different risks from cancer and genetic effects to the tissue that was irradiated. It is well known that different tissues have different sensitivities to these stochastic effects. For example, the breast seems to be relatively sensitive to the induction of cancer, whereas other tissues and organs are far less sensitive. The effective dose equivalent attempts to account for these differences in risk between organs. It is important to note that this term applies only when exposure occurs from external sources.

Committed Dose Equivalent

Committed dose equivalent is the term used when incorporated radionuclides are the source of exposure. The NCRP defines this as the dose equivalent over 50 years following the intake of a radionuclide. Fifty years has been chosen since it corresponds to the working life of an individual.

Genetically Significant Dose (GSD)

To evaluate the genetic impact of these low doses on the whole population, the term Genetic Significant Dose (GSD) is used. This is an average figure calculated from the actual gonadal doses received by the exposed population, which also takes into account the expected contribution of these individuals to children in future generations. It is assumed that this dose, received by every member of the population, would have the same genetic effect as the doses that are now being received by the segment of the population exposed to medical and/or dental x-rays.

DIAGNOSTIC RADIOLOGY

Exposure Facts

The use of x-rays for diagnostic purposes has increased dramatically in the last 20 years (see Table 9–2). This use is not restricted to any one age group (Table 9–3), although the majority of exams are per-

*Sievert (Sv) is the new SI unit; 1 rem = 0.01 Sv.

formed in the over-40 age group for obvious age-related health reasons. Even though the dose to a patient from any one particular exam has steadily decreased over this same time, the fact that so many people—about one-half of the population each year—are exposed to ionizing radiation is of concern.

Radiation doses to individuals and to the general population for some common diagnostic x-ray procedures are given in Table 9–4 for 1980. Estimated total body doses, gonadal doses, and doses to the embryo from some common diagnostic procedures are given in Table 9–5.

Carcinogenesis

It has been shown that radiation does, indeed, cause cancer, particularly in sensitive tissues such as breast, thyroid gland, and bone marrow (see Chapter 8). Leukemia is one cancer frequently associated with radiation. Studies of circulating lymphocytes of patients at various times following diagnostic x-ray procedures have shown that the numbers and types of chromosome breaks increase with increasing dose. Skin exposures of 20 mR to 3 R produce no chromosome abnormalities in circulating lymphocytes. Doses of this magnitude are given during examinations such as chest radiographs and intravenous pyelograms (IVPs). However, chromosome fragments have been observed in the lymphocytes of patients who have undergone cardiac catheterization, a procedure that results in exposures of 4 R to 12 R and higher. Upper GI and barium enema (BE) procedures that may give doses up to 35 mR, produce both simple and complex aberrations (e.g., fragments, dicentrics, and rings) in the chromosomes of circulating lymphocytes.

TABLE 9–3.

Distribution of X-ray and Nuclear Medicine Examinations Among Various Age Groups in the U.S. Population in 1980*

Age range	Percent of U.S. Population in Age Group	Percent of Age Group Receiving	
		X-ray Examinations (Mettler, 1987)	Nuclear Medicine Examinations (Mettler et al, 1982)
<15	23	10	2
15–29	27	21	8
30–44	19	17	14
45–64	20	27	37
>64	11	26	39

*From National Council on Radiation Protection and Measurements: *Ionizing Radiation Exposure of the Population of the United States.* Washington DC, US Government Printing Office, NCRPM Report No 93, 1987. Used by permission.

TABLE 9-4.

Collective Effective Dose Equivalent for the U.S. in 1980 From Diagnostic Medical X-ray Examinations*

Examination	Annual Number of Examinations (thousands)	Average Effective Dose Equivalent per Examination (μSv)‡	Annual Collective Effective Dose Equivalent† (person-Sv)§
Computed tomography (head and body)	3,300	1,100	3,700
Chest	64,000	60	4,100
Skull and other head and neck	8,200	200	1,800
Cervical spine	5,100	200	1,000
Biliary tract	3,400	1,900	6,400
Lumbar spine	12,900	1,300	16,400
Upper GI tract	7,600	2,450	18,500
Kidney, ureters, bladder	7,900	550	4,400
Barium enema	4,900	4,050	19,900
Intravenous pyelogram	4,200	1,600	6,600
Pelvis and hip	4,700	650	3,000
Extremities	45,000	10	450
Other¶	8,400	500	4,200
Rounded total	**180,000**	**500**	**~91,000**

*From National Council on Radiation Protection and Measurement: *Ionizing Radiation Exposure of the Population of the United States.* Washington DC, US Government Printing Office Report No. 93, 1987. Used by permission.
†Numbers obtained from product of two previous columns but using unrounded figures.
‡μSv = 0.1 mrem.
§1 person-Sv = 100 person-rem.
¶Estimated from the average of all examinations.

TABLE 9-5.

Total Body and Organ Doses From Some Common Diagnostic X-ray Procedure (in mrem)*

Examination	Total-Body	Testes	Ovaries	Embryo
Chest	8–11	—	—	—
Kidneys	29–57	15	210	260
Barium enema	130–260	60	790	820
Lumbosacral spine	119–231	45	640	640
IVP	82–158	50	640	820
Hip	11–21	370	80	130
Pelvis	19–36	55	150	200
Upper GI	138–231	—	45	50

*From American College of Radiology: *Medical Radiation: A Guide to Good Practice.* Chicago, ACR Committee on Radiological Units, Standards and Protection, 1985. Used by permission.

Although the health impact of these mutations in circulating lymphocytes is difficult to evaluate, the question certainly arises of the later development of leukemia. Radiation *is* a known causative agent for leukemia (Chapter 8), but the role of diagnostic radiology in the etiology of the disease remains speculative. Some investigators believe that, particularly in procedures that result in higher radiation doses, mutations probably have occurred in stem cells resulting in a continual propagation of these mutations in circulating lymphocytes. Whether these mutated cells eventually produce leukemia is unknown. At the present time, there is no conclusive evidence that doses from diagnostic examinations pose any hazard to adult patients in terms of leukemia. Nonetheless, because so many are exposed, it is reasonable to attempt to estimate the number of leukemias and other cancers that might be induced by the doses from these diagnostic x-ray procedures.

Hall has estimated that the number of leukemias that might be induced by diagnostic x-rays in 1 year is from 218 to 712, and that about 1,000 cancers per year of all sorts might arise from the diagnostic uses of radiation. Although this might seem to represent a large risk, it must be remembered that about *one million* new cancers arise spontaneously in the population each year! The cancer risk from diagnostic x-ray procedures is very small. Nonetheless, if you are one of the potential 1,000 people at risk for radiation-induced cancer, the number of other people with cancer is not important. For the individual, even this small risk of cancer induction might contraindicate the use of x-rays for diagnostic reasons. The critical issue is, What is the benefit of such procedures vs. these risks? Clearly, the benefits of a speedy diagnosis of a medical problem followed by prompt treatment outweigh this small probability of cancer years later.

However, this same reasoning does not apply to the use of x-rays for routine screening. This is particularly true for mammograms. The breast appears to be exquisitely sensitive to radiation. Thus, although routine mammograms are critical for women who are identified as at a high risk for breast cancer, they are not necessary for the majority of women and, if used indiscriminately in all women, particularly in young women, this procedure may in fact *induce* as many tumors as it detects!

The same argument applies to the use of dental x-ray examinations. A full dental series can give as much as 0.05 Gy to the oral cavity. If given twice a year at each check-up, this amounts to 0.10 Gy. The tissue at risk is the thyroid, another sensitive tissue to the induction of cancer. It is likely that a number of cancers are induced by these dental exposures, particularly since half the population see their dentist each year. The indiscriminate use of dental x-rays should be discouraged, particularly for children.

Genetic Risks

The harm to future generations is of concern in diagnostic radiology. The genetic risks from medical diagnostic x-ray procedures are even more difficult to assess than the risk of cancer induction. In this situation the risk is not to the individual receiving the exam, but to that person's offspring, particularly in the first two generations after exposure. Because radiation-induced mutations are nonthreshold, they are usually considered to be detrimental, and they may be exhibited in generations long after exposure has occurred. The dose received by the gonads from diagnostic examinations is important. Table 9–5 shows that many routine diagnostic exams deliver relatively large doses to the gonads of men and women. For this reason alone, genetic effects become important.

One way to attempt to estimate the genetic risks is to compare the genetic significant dose (GSD) from such procedures with the doubling dose (see Chapter 8). The GSD from diagnostic x-rays is estimated at 20 to 30 mrem, whereas the doubling dose is 50 to 250 mrem—clearly well above the estimated GSD. For this reason alone, it is unlikely that diagnostic x-rays will change the incidence of mutations. Also, the 20 to 30 mrem contribution to the GSD from diagnostic x-rays is far less than that from natural background sources (see Table 9–1). As long as this trend continues, i.e., the GSD from natural sources is higher than from medical exposures, there is little reason to worry about genetic changes from the medical use of x-rays.

Based on these statistics, Hall has estimated that the number of genetic disorders produced per year by medical radiation range from 143 to 3,564. This must be compared to the 368,000 per year that arise naturally in the United States population.

It appears then that the risks associated with diagnostic x-rays is small. However, x-rays should not be used indiscriminately. No medical radiation is justified *unless the benefit outweighs the risk*. It is imperative that gonadal exposure be kept to a minimum during all diagnostic procedures and that all precautions be taken to ensure that the gonads receive no unnecessary exposure. Gonadal shields should always be used when the gonadal area is not of interest in the study; the use of shields decreases gonadal doses by 90%. The avoidance of unnecessary repeat exposures would decrease the GSD by 10%, and an additional 30% decrease would result from improved technique. In general, a 50% decrease in GSD could be achieved with improved technique and education. It has been estimated that proper collimation alone (collimating the x-ray beam so that the beam is no larger than the film) would reduce the GSD by 65%.

Risks to the Embryo and Fetus

It is well known that the embryo and fetus are exquisitely sensitive to ionizing radiation (see Chapter 7). Although conclusive evidence implicates radiation in the production of many congenital abnormalities, the deforming effects on the fetus of doses from diagnostic procedures remain controversial, as does the evidence concerning the induction of leukemia and other childhood malignancies (Chapter 8).

Estimated radiation doses to the fetus for some diagnostic procedures are given in Table 9–5. Another method of estimating fetal doses is by the dose delivered to the ovaries. The range of estimated doses to the ovaries from some common x-ray procedures is given in Table 9–6. It is suggested that the dose to an unsuspected embryo could be 25% higher than the values in the table, which would be significant in the high-dose group. That these doses can cause changes in the embryo can be appreciated from Table 9–7, which gives observed chromosome mutations in the fetus as a result of irradiation in utero.

The major problem arising from exposure of the fetus to diagnostic x-rays is that the most radiosensitive period in the life of the fetus is the first 6 weeks, when a woman is usually unaware of her pregnancy. Doses as low as 10 rad (0.10 Gy) are believed harmful to the fetus during the first 6 weeks of gestation. As a result, it is recommended that the possibility of pregnancy be ruled out in all female patients between the ages of 11 to 50 prior to administering diagnostic procedures involving radiation and that the "10-day rule" be followed. This rule, suggested by the National Commission on Radiation Protection and Measurement (NCRP), recommends that all nonemergency diagnostic procedures involving the pelvis in women of childbearing age be conducted during the first 10 days of the menstrual cycle, when the probability of pregnancy is very small.

Because of this recommendation, many radiologists in both private practice and in hospitals have initiated "elective booking" procedures to identify the potentially pregnant patient. This involves obtaining a menstrual history on all female patients between the ages of 11 and 50, and booking patients considered nonemergencies during the first 10 days of their menstrual cycles. Of course, diagnostic examinations are performed on patients who are considered to have emergencies at any time, regardless of menstrual cycle.

What should be done if a woman discovers she is pregnant after receiving a series of pelvic x-rays? This is a potentially drastic situation as exposure will have occurred during the time when the fetus was extremely sensitive to radiation. For these reasons, some recommend

TABLE 9–6.

Estimated Dose to the Ovaries (Uterus) Expressed in Millirads per Radiographic Examination*†

Type of Examination	Estimated Mean Dose from Bureau of Radiological Health Report‡	Reported Range of Doses
Low-dose group		
Dental	0.03–0.1	0.03–0.1
Head, cervical spine	<0.5	<0.5–3
Extremities	<0.5	<0.5–18
Shoulder	<0.5	<0.5–3
Thoracic spine	11	<10–55
Chest (radiographic)	1	0.2–43
Chest (photofluorographic)	3	0.9–40
Moderate-dose group		
Upper GI series	171	5–1,230
Cholecystography	78	14–1,600
Cholangiography		
High-dose group†		
Lumbar spine	721	20–2,900
Lumbosacral spine		
Pelvis	210	40–1,600
Hip and femur (proximal)	124	53–1,000
Urography, IV, or retrograde pyelogram	588	50–4,000
Urethrocystography		200–3,000
Lower GI tract (barium enema)	903	20–9,200
Abdomen	221	18–1,400
Abdomen (obstetric)		110–1,600
Pelvimetry		160–4,000
Hysterosalpingography		200–6,700

*From *Medical Radiation Exposure of Pregnant and Potentially Pregnant Women,* National Council on Radiation Protection and Measurements. Report 54, Bethesda, MD, 1979.
†Figures are dose estimates to the ovaries for the complete radiographic examination, but not including fluoroscopy. The actual doses to the embryo (uterus) in group C would be expected to be typically 25% to 50% greater than the tabulated dose for ovaries (Rosenstein, 1976). The use of fluoroscopy could further increase the dose to the embryo by appreciable amounts.
‡The upper limits in the ranges shown are the maximum reported in the cited literature and, therefore, in most cases are much higher than the expected dose to the embryo-fetus for an average-sized woman when current standards of good radiological practice are followed. The mean values given in column 2 (BRH) are probably the best estimate of mean ovarian doses in the United States at the present time. See BRH (1976) for a more detailed report on the distribution of doses to the ovaries.

an abortion if the embryo receives 10 rad (0.10 Gy) during the first 6 weeks of gestation.

To put this into perspective, Hall has calculated that a dose of 1 rad (0.01 Gy) given in utero would add, on average, two additional malformations to the 60 that occur naturally in every 1,000 births per year. Thus the risk is very small, indeed. Nonetheless, every effort should be made to ensure that a fetus is not unknowingly irradiated. Again, however, the risk versus the benefit must be a compelling factor in this decision.

NUCLEAR MEDICINE

Radiopharmaceuticals have been used in the diagnosis and treatment of disease since 1946 and, therefore, are relative newcomers to the medical uses of radiation. Today the specialty of nuclear medicine is a dynamic, growing, and vital area of medicine with new radiopharmaceuticals and diverse applications of these materials being developed constantly, as well as new and improved instrumentation.

Although the percentage of the population exposed to radiation via nuclear medicine procedures is low in comparison to diagnostic radiology, the health impact of these procedures is still of concern. As in diagnostic radiology, nuclear medicine procedures result in low radiation doses, the potential biologic risks of which are carcinogenic (particularly leukemia) and genetic effects. Those groups at risk include patients, personnel, fetuses, and future generations.

Exposure Facts

Both the diagnostic and therapeutic uses of radiopharmaceuticals are dependent on the accumulation of the material in the target organ, i.e., the organ of interest. Some radiopharmaceuticals have an affinity for certain organs that are not necessarily the organ of interest; these

TABLE 9–7.

Chromosome Mutation in Fetuses Exposed in Utero During Diagnostic Radiographic and Fluoroscopic Procedures*

Case Number	Estimated Dose or Exposure	Type of Examination	Fetal Age at Exposure (Weeks)	Tissue Studied	Chromosome Mutations
1	0.19 rad	Abdominal hyster-osalpingography	10–11	—	None
2	3.0 R	—	6	Skin, lung	Translocations and others
3	3.9 rad	Barium meal, enema	6	Chorionic fragments	Deletions, dicentrics
4	—	Radiopelvimetry	1	Lymphocytes, fibroblasts	Extra chromosome markers

*From Dalrymple GV, et al: *Medical Radiation Biology*. Philadelphia, WB Saunders, 1973. Used by permission.

organs are termed "critical organs." The critical organ is that organ which, although it may not accumulate the greatest amount of the radiopharmaceutical, dictates the amount of a radiopharmaceutical that can be administered. This amount is based not only on the accumulation in the organ, but, more importantly, on the radiation sensitivity of the organ. The critical organ is therefore the dose-limiting factor in a radiopharmaceutical procedure. Because the determination of biologic effect and health risk to the patient is dependent on the amount of radiation received, the critical organ is of primary importance. However, radiopharmaceuticals are transported throughout the body by the bloodstream, resulting in exposure to the total body, which is also of concern. Table 9–8 lists the exposure to critical organs and total body from widely used radiopharmaceuticals.

Two general factors are considered when estimating patient exposure in nuclear medicine: physical and biologic. The physical factors, e.g., the type of radiation emitted, energy, and physical half-life, are well defined. The biologic variables are less well defined and, unfortunately, play a significant role in determining radiation exposure to the individual, thereby contributing greatly to uncertainties in exposure estimations. These biologic variables result in problems in determining exposure in nuclear medicine, particularly in terms of the patient, unique from those encountered in other medical uses of radiation.

Biologic Variables

The biologic effect of a radionuclide is dependent on both its physical and biologic half-life, the latter being a function of the rate at which the nuclide is metabolized and eliminated from the body. Less is known concerning the biologic half-lives than the well-defined physical half-lives. Unfortunately, the biologic half-life is the main determinant of radiation exposure in an organ, because this factor determines the amount of time the radiopharmaceutical remains in the organ.

One biologic factor that plays a large role is the fact that most patients undergoing nuclear medicine procedure are ill. The critical organ values listed in Table 9–8 represent exposures in healthy individuals. These figures, which may vary widely even among healthy persons, may be changed to an even greater extent by the presence of disease in the organ. Disease may affect the size or the function of the organ, thus influencing the amount of radionuclide accumulated, which in turn alters the radiation exposure to the critical organ. In addition, exposure to secondary organs that accumulate the radionuclide may be changed.

TABLE 9–8.
Radiation Doses for Selected Nuclear Medicine Procedures*

Radiopharmaceuticals	Study	Age (years)†	Mean Dose (mrad/µCi administered)‡						
			Gonads		Kidneys	Marrow (red)	Spleen	Thyroid	Total-Body
			Testes	Ovaries					
51Cr-chromate red cells	Red cell survival time or volume	A	0.23	0.29		0.31	14		0.28
57Co-vitamin B-12	Vitamin B-12 absorption	A	1.1	1.6		2			10
67Ga-citrate	Tumor and abscess imaging	A	0.26		0.41	0.58	0.6		0.16
		10	0.44				1		0.28
		1	0.93				2.6		0.57
		N	2.6				8		1.4
99mTc DTPA	Renal imaging (dynamic)	A	0.020	0.027	0.085	0.010			0.016
		10	0.110	0.049	0.144				0.029
		1	0.132	0.110	0.318				0.062
		N	0.170	0.330	0.828				0.170
99mTc-glucoheptonate	Renal imaging	A	0.0038	0.0069	0.3	0.012			0.01
99mTc-macroaggregates	Perfusion study	A	0.007	0.009	0.16	0.015	0.017	0.008	0.015
		10	0.038	0.016					0.028
		1	0.046	0.038					0.064
		N	0.06	0.11					0.18
99mTc-pertechnetate	Thyroid imaging	A	0.012	0.017		0.022		0.20	0.013
	Thyroid imaging	10	0.066	0.032				0.48	0.024
	or ectopic gastric mucosa imaging	1	0.079	0.076				1.3	0.055
		N	0.1	0.22				3.4	0.15
99mTc-pyrophosphate, methylene diphosphate	Bone imaging	A	0.015	0.015	0.03	0.035			0.013
99mTc-red blood cells	Blood pool imaging	A	0.012	0.021	0.03	0.023	0.018	0.041	0.017

99mTc-sulfur colloid	Liver, spleen, bone marrow imaging	A	0.019	0.023		0.027 (nl)	0.21 (nl)		0.019
						0.045 (e,i)	0.28 (e,i)		0.018
						0.079 (i,d)	0.42 (i,d)		0.016
		10	0.1	0.014			0.6		0.027
		1	0.13	0.097			1.2		0.056
		N	0.16	0.28			2.7		0.14
113mIn-DTPA	Brain imaging (static and dynamic)	A	0.005	0.009	1.9	0.011			0.01
		10							0.015
		1							0.04
		N							0.13
123I-iodide	Thyroid imaging	A	0.025	0.034		0.044		2.4	0.03
		10	0.051					30	0.051
		1	0.12					110	0.13
		N	0.35					160	0.35
201Ti-chloride	Myocardial imaging	A	0.52	0.47	1.2			0.64	0.21

*Modified from Hall EJ: *Radiobiology for the Radiologist*, ed 3. Philadelphia, JB Lippincott, 1988.

†A, adult; N, newborn.

‡nl, normal liver; e,i, early to intermediate diffuse parenchymal disease; i,d, intermediate to advanced diffuse parenchymal disease.

TABLE 9–9.

Body Weights and Organ Weights for Various Ages*

| | Weight (g) | | | | | |
Organ	Newborn	1 year	5 years	10 years	15 years	Adult
Whole-body	3,540.	12,100.	20,300.	33,500.	55,000.	70,000
Thyroid	1.9	2.5	6.1	8.7	15.8	20
Kidney	23.0	72.0	112.0	187.0	247.0	300
Liver	136.0	333.0	591.0	918.0	1,289.0	1,700
Spleen	9.4	31.0	54.0	101.0	138.0	150

*From Kereiakes J, et al: Patient and personnel dose during radioisotope procedures, in *Medical Radiation Information for Litigation,* Proceedings of a Conference, Baylor University College of Medicine, Houston, November 21–22, 1968. Washington DC, US Government Printing Office, Publication No DMRE 69-3, 1969. Used by permission.

A second major problem is the age of the patient. Physiologic processes, metabolic rate and organ sizes in children differ from those in adults, and even vary between infants and children (Table 9–9). Any one or a combination of these factors can result in an alteration in the uptake of radionuclide in the body and the exposure to various organs. Table 9–10 presents the doses received by organs in children from various radionuclides. Note the change in dose from each radionuclide as a function of age; in all cases, the dose decreases with increasing age. Although lower doses are given to children undergoing nuclear medicine procedures, many questions remain concerning the fate of these materials in the body. Unlike adults, where a "standard" or "reference" person is used for exposure calculations, a "standard" child has not been established. In all likelihood, based on the information in Tables 9–9 and 9–10, there will have to be at least two standards for children: one for infants and one for older children.

As in diagnostic radiology, the potential health impact on the general population from incorporated radionuclides is of concern. The collective effective dose equivalents from some common diagnostic nuclear medicine tests are shown in Table 9–11. An interesting point is that over 50% of the collective effective dose equivalent comes from brain, bone, and cardiovascular exams. As with diagnostic radiology, the question now is, What do these numbers represent in terms of the health-related risks?

Carcinogenesis

More than 40 years' experience has revealed no significant adverse effects from these procedures in terms of later-appearing cancers. In general, diagnostic nuclear medicine procedures are believed to pose

TABLE 9–10.

Absorbed Dose to Critical Organs for Selected Radiopharmaceuticals*

Radionuclide	Pharmaceutical	Critical Organ	Critical Organ Dose (mrad/μCi administered)				
			Newborn	1 year	5 years	15 years	Adult
^{51}Cr	RBC (heat-treated)	Spleen	336.00	90.10	56.20	24.10	22.50
^{67}Ga	Citrate	Spleen	8.02	2.60	1.64	0.71	0.60
^{99m}Tc	DTPA	Bladder†	5.00	1.70	1.10	0.56	0.45
		Kidney	0.39	0.15	0.10	0.05	0.04
	HIDA	Liver	0.79	0.37	0.25	0.11	0.09
	HSA	Blood	0.81	0.24	0.15	0.06	0.05
	Iron complex	Renal cortex	5.20	1.80	1.20	0.61	0.55
	MAA (microspheres)	Lung	3.09	1.00	0.59	0.26	0.20
	Pertechnetate	LLI‡	1.91	0.67	0.46	0.23	0.20
	Polyphosphate	Bone	1.10	0.32	0.23	0.10	0.08
	RBC (heat treated)	Spleen	26.00	9.23	5.21	2.70	2.60
	Sulfur colloid	Liver	2.90	1.34	0.92	0.40	0.33
^{111}In	Iron hydroxide	Lung	14.70	4.45	2.50	1.11	0.77
	Colloid	Liver	107.33	47.70	27.77	12.61	10.60
	DTPA	Bladder^a	24.60	7.45	4.43	1.89	1.48
^{123}I	Iodohippurate	Kidney	0.69	0.23	0.18	0.10	0.07
	Rose bengal	Liver	1.89	0.75	0.46	0.25	0.20
^{131}I	Hippuran	Kidney	9.52	4.44	3.08	1.20	1.00
	HSA	Blood	309.50	92.50	55.50	20.80	16.00
	MAA	Lung	73.80	22.20	13.10	5.60	4.00
	Rose bengal	Liver	8.10	3.00	1.77	0.84	0.67

*From National Council on Radiation Protection and Measurements: *Protection in Nuclear Medicine and Ultrasound Diagnostic Procedures in Children.* Washington, DC, US Government Printing Office, NCRNM Report No 73, 1983. Used by permission.

†Assumes 6-hour bladder residence time.

‡Perchlorate blocking dose (IV administration)

no more hazard to the patient than are diagnostic radiology procedures, and are not considered to deliver excessive radiation doses. In fact, patient exposures from nuclear medicine are usually lower than those from radiography. From the evidence available, the risk of inducing cancers in adult patients from diagnostic nuclear medicine procedures is very small—on the same order as the risk of cancer induction from radiography. Hall estimates that such procedures could induce up to 80 leukemias and a total of 300 new cancers per year. When compared with the one million new cancer cases that arise spontaneously in one year, the risk from nuclear medicine procedures constitutes the proverbial drop in the bucket.

Genetic Risks

Gonadal doses from various radiopharmaceuticals are listed in Table 9–8. In 1970 the GSD from nuclear medicine was estimated to be 0.3 mR; compared with the GSD from diagnostic radiology (20 mR), the former is relatively minor. This low contribution to the GSD is due to two factors. Until 1970 only a small proportion of the general population was exposed to nuclear medicine procedures. The estimated 20% increase in the use of radiopharmaceuticals for diagnostic purposes will gradually result in exposure of a larger number of individuals. In

TABLE 9–11.

Collective Effective Dose Equivalent From Diagnostic Nuclear Medicine Tests in the U.S. in 1982*

Examination	Annual Number of Examinations (thousands)	Average Effective Dose Equivalent per Examination (μSv)[‡]	Average Annual Collective Effective Dose Equivalent[†] (person-Sv)[§]
Brain	810	6,500	5,300
Hepatobiliary	180	3,700	700
Liver	1,400	2,400	3,400
Bone	1,800	4,400	8,000
Lung	1,200	1,500	1,800
Thyroid	680	5,900	4,000
Kidney	240	3,100	700
Tumor	120	12,000	1,500
Cardiovascular	950	7,100	6,700
Rounded Total	**7,400**	**4,300**	**32,000**

*From National Council on Radiation Protection and Measurements: *Ionizing Radiation Exposure of the Population of the United States,* Washington DC, US Government Printing Office, NCRPM Report No 93, 1987. Used by permission.
†Number obtained from product of previous two columns but using unrounded figures.
‡1 μSv = 0.1 mrem.
§1 person-Sv = 100 person-rem.

addition, in the past a large segment of the potential child-bearing individuals—the genetically significant population—were not exposed to nuclear medicine procedures because of the warning that radiopharmaceuticals were absolutely contraindicated in persons under 18 years of age. This factor also is changing as larger numbers of children are receiving radiopharmaceuticals for diagnostic purposes.

Because of the changing trends in the administration of radionuclides to these persons, particularly the increased use in persons under the age of 18, nuclear medicine will contribute a larger percentage of the GSD in the next few years. Comparing the GSD from nuclear medicine, ~2 mrems, with that from natural background radiation, >25 mrems, it is clear that the same arguments and conclusions apply as in diagnostic radiology, i.e., as long as the GSD from these procedures is less than that from background radiation, the genetic load of such procedures is very small. Based on the figures, Hall estimates that 12 to 226 extra mutations could be induced by nuclear medicine procedures.

Effects on Children and the Fetus

The risks to children from diagnostic nuclear medicine procedures are more difficult to evaluate. Based on the fact that children are generally more sensitive to radiation than are adults, and that many physiologic and metabolic factors concerning radionuclide use in children are unknown, doses from diagnostic procedures may pose more of a hazard to children than to adults.

Even less clear is the risk to the fetus. Table 9–12 shows absorbed doses to the embryo for some selected nuclear medicine procedures. Table 9–13 shows the dose to the fetal thyroid of ^{131}I given to the mother at various gestational stages. Because of the sensitivity of fetal tissues, biologic damage could occur. The biggest concern has always been the potential to increase the incidence of childhood cancers from such procedures. However, studies of the children irradiated in utero in Japan during the atomic bombing have shown no increase in childhood cancers. Nonetheless, physicians are, and perhaps should be even more, cautious in the use of radionuclides in a pregnant or potentially pregnant woman than they are in diagnostic radiology, even though the doses may be similar.

Table 9–14 summarizes the important exposure doses to the bone marrow and the gonads from diagnostic x-rays and nuclear medicine. Dental examinations have been omitted because their contribution is minimal.

TABLE 9–12.

Estimated Absorbed Dose to Embryo for Selected
Radiopharmaceuticals*

Radiopharmaceutical	Embryo Absorbed Dose (rad/mCi administered)
^{99m}Tc (various procedures)	0.18–0.40
^{123}Sodium iodide (15% uptake)	0.032
^{131}I Sodium iodide (15% uptake)	0.100
^{123}I Rose bengal	0.130
^{131}I Rose bengal	0.680

*From National Council on Radiation Protection and Measurements: *Protection in Nuclear Medicine and Ultrasound Diagnostic Procedures in Children,* Washington DC, US Government Printing Office, NCRPM Report No 73, 1983. Used by permission.

TABLE 9–13.

Absorbed Dose to Fetal Thyroid Gland From Administered to the Mother ^{131}I*

Gestation Period	Fetal/Maternal Ratio (thyroid gland)[†]	Absorbed Dose to Fetal Thyroid (rad/μCi)[‡]
10–12 wks	—	0.001 (precursors)
12–13 wks	1.2	0.7
2nd trimester	1.8	6.0
3rd trimester	7.5	—
Birth imminent	—	8.0

*From National Council on Radiation Protection and Measurements: *Protection in Nuclear Medicine and Ultrasound Diagnostic Procedures in Children.* Washington DC, US Government Printing Office. NCRPM Report No 73, 1983. Used by permission.
[†]μCi/g
[‡]rad/μCi of ^{131}I ingested by mother.

Therapeutic Use of Radionuclides

Radionuclides are used in the treatment of hyperthyroidism and thyroid carcinoma using ^{131}I.

The use of ^{131}I in the treatment of hyperthyroidism has been a successful means of controlling this disease for many years. However, as with any use of radiation for medical purposes, the issue is whether this treatment carries any risk with it, particularly in terms of leukemia and the later development of thyroid carcinoma. There is no question that radiation can induce thyroid carcinoma. There is an increased incidence of thyroid carcinoma in children irradiated for enlarged thymus glands, an increased incidence of thyroid carcinoma in children irradiated for tinea capitis (ring worm), and an increased incidence of thyroid carcinomas has been found in the Marshall Islanders exposed to fallout radiation.

In contrast to these rather conclusive data, an increased incidence of thyroid cancer *has not been observed* in the adult population after treatment of hyperthyroidism with ^{131}I. The discrepancy between these data and those from the children and Marshall Islander experiences is most likely due to the fact that the treatment of hyperthyroidism requires much higher doses of radiation than were received in the other situations. These high doses are of the magnitude that will kill cells, thus these cells do not survive the treatment and, therefore, do not proliferate and express other types of radiation-induced damage, such as cancer, in the future. This reasoning is supported by the observation that years after treatment for hyperthyroidism, patients are hypothyroid—their thyroid glands are smaller, indicating that cells have been killed, resulting in an atrophied gland.

Previously, ^{131}I therapy for hyperthyroidism was not used on persons under 40 years of age, although this age limit has been decreased to 20 years. Although there is no evidence that ^{131}I induces thyroid carcinoma in adults, a sufficient time period has not yet elapsed to evaluate the results of this therapy on the thyroid in children and adolescents.

TABLE 9–14.

Effective Dose Equivalents From Medical Exposures in 1980*

Modality and Target Tissue	Annual Collective Effective Dose Equivalent (thousand person-rems)	Average Annual Effective Dose Equivalent to the U.S. Population (mrems)
Diagnostic x-rays		
GSD		
Male	—	4–10
Female	—	18–20
Total	5,000–6,900	22–30
Bone marrow	16,000–25,000	74–114
Total effective dose equivalent	9,050–13,000	39 (25–55)
Nuclear medicine		
GSD	440	1.9
Bone marrow	3,200	14
Total effective dose equivalent	3,200	14

*From National Council on Radiation Protection and Measurements: *Exposure of the Population in the United States to Ionizing Radiation.* Washington DC, US Government Printing Office, NCRPM Report No 93, 1987. Used by permission.

The treatment of hyperthyroidism with ^{131}I has been associated with occasional leukemia in some patients. The study of patients treated for hyperthyroidism with ^{131}I revealed a slight increase of leukemia in this population when compared with the general population. However, hyperthyroid patients treated by surgery alone also showed the same increased leukemia incidence. A study has now been completed of a large number of patients (36,000) from a number of medical centers in the United States under the auspices of the U.S. Bureau of Radiological Health. The results of this study showed that there *is not* an increased incidence of leukemia in hyperthyroid patients treated with ^{131}I. Interestingly, however, it was found that patients with hyperthyroidism itself have an enhanced risk of leukemia regardless of the treatment. Based on these data, then, it is most likely that ^{131}I treatment for hyperthyroidism carries no measurable risk of leukemia, although certainly one cannot say with certainty that there is no risk.

An absolute contraindication to the treatment of hyperthyroidism with ^{131}I is pregnancy. Iodine crosses the placenta barrier and localizes in the fetal thyroid, particularly after the first trimester, necessitating another form of treatment.

OCCUPATIONAL EXPOSURES

It is estimated that about 1.5 million people are employed in radiation-related work. This figure includes those employed in the medical field, as well as those employed in industry, including nuclear power plant workers. Table 9–15 shows the number of persons employed and the effective and collective effective dose equivalents to the various workers.

Occupationally exposed personnel present a different problem than do patients. In contrast to patients who are exposed to medical/dental radiation relatively few times during their lifetimes, workers in radiation are exposed to chronic low doses throughout their professional lives. Chromosome mutations in circulating lymphocytes are much more frequent in occupationally exposed individuals, increasing with the number of years employed. Figure 9–2 shows the chromosomes from a cell taken from a radiologist whose lymphocytes had a number of chromosome mutations. Although historically radiation workers were at a very high risk for cancer induction, the increased incidence of cancers in occupationally exposed individuals has disappeared. This decreased cancer incidence is directly attributable to the establishment of and reduction in the Maximum Permissible Dose (MPD).

TABLE 9–15.

Exposure of Radiation Workers to Low-LET Radiation for 1980*

Occupational Category	Number of Workers (thousands)		Average Annual Effective Dose Equivalent (mSv)†		Collective Effective Dose Equivalent (person-Sv)‡
	All	Exposed	All	Exposed	
Medicine	584	277	0.7	1.5	410
Industry	305	156	1.2	2.4	380
Nuclear fuel cycle	151	91	3.6	6.0	540
Government	204	105	0.6	1.2	120
Miscellaneous	76	31	0.7	1.6	50
Other workers	115	107	1.7	1.8	200
Others (e.g., visitors)	155	42	0.25	0.9	40
Rounded subtotal	**1,590**	**810**	**1.1**	**2.1**	**1,700**

*From National Council on Radiation Protection and Measurements: *Ionizing Radiation Exposure of the Population of the United States.* Washington DC, US Government Printing Office, NCRPM Report No 93, 1987. Used by permission.
†1 mSv = 100 mrem.
‡1 person-Sv = 100 person-rem.

The Concept of Maximum Permissible Dose

Recognition of the harmful effects of radiation and the biologic risk involved resulted in the establishment of limitations on the amount of radiation received by all individuals, including the general population and occupationally exposed persons.

The rationale for MPDs is that, although there is no tolerance to radiation, there is an acceptable risk for occupationally exposed persons. The present limits are within this risk, because from the evidence available there does not appear to be excess danger to occupationally exposed personnel from radiation—provided, of course, that all rules and regulations of radiation hygiene are followed.

Imposed in the 1920s, these limits have been constantly reduced, reflecting the realization that there is no dose below which the risk of radiation damage is nonexistent (i.e., no threshold dose). Originally termed Tolerance Doses, then Maximum Permissible Doses, the current philosophy is that the dose should be kept "as low as reasonably achievable" (ALRA).

The NCRP currently recommends the following:

1. Five rem should remain as the *maximum* permissible dose equivalent for total-body exposure. The key word here is *maximum*; this is the upper boundary, and all efforts should be made to stay well below this figure.

2. Previously, exposed individuals could receive a total-body exposure of 5 rem/year after the age of 18. The NCRP now recommends that this be discontinued.
3. Instead, the cumulative exposure for an occupationally exposed person should not exceed his age in years times 1 rem.
4. In the exposure of pregnant women under occupational conditions, the limit for the fetus is 5 rem, which should not be received at a rate greater than 0.05 rem/month.
5. All limits include the sum of internal and external exposures.

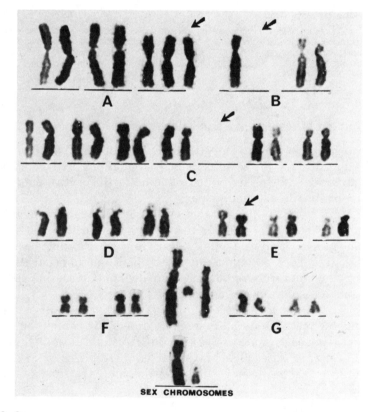

SEX CHROMOSOMES

FIG 9–2.
Chromosome damage in the lymphocyte of a long-practicing radiologist. *Arrows* indicate various types of damage. A dicentric chromosome and two acentric fragments are seen between *F* and *G*. There was a 7% incidence of chromosome mutations compared to 2% mutations in the nonoccupationally exposed control. (From Dalrymple GV, et al: *Medical Radiation Biology.* Philadelphia, WB Saunders, 1973, p 75. Used by permission.)

TABLE 9–16.

Summary of Recommendations*†

Type of Exposure	Dose	
	mSv	rem
A. Occupational exposures (annual)‡		
1. Effective dose equivalent limit (stochastic effects)	50 mSv	5 rem
2. Dose equivalent limits for tissues and organs (nonstochastic effects)		
a. Lens of eye	150 mSv	15 rem
b. All others (e.g., red bone marrow, breast, lung, gonads, skin, and extremities)	500 mSv	50 rem
3. Guidance: Cumulative exposure	10 mSv × age	1 rem × age in years
B. Public exposures (annual)		
1. Effective dose equivalent limit, continuous or frequent exposure‡	1 mSv	0.1 rem
2. Effective dose equivalent limit, infrequent exposure‡	5 mSv	0.5 rem
3. Remedial action recommended when:		
a. Effective dose equivalent§	>5 mSv	>0.5 rem
4. Dose equivalent limits for lens of eye	50 mSv	5 rem
C. Education and training exposures (annual)‡		
1. Effective dose equivalent limit	1 mSv	0.1 rem
2. Dose equivalent limit for lens of eye, skin, and extremities	50 mSv	5 rem
D. Embryo-fetus exposures†		
1. Total dose equivalent limit	5 mSv	0.5 rem
2. Dose equivalent limit in a month	0.5 mSv	0.05 rem

*From National Council on Radiation Protection and Measurements: *Recommendations on Limits for Exposure to Ionizing Radiation.* Washington DC, US Government Printing Office, NCRPM Report No 91, 1987. Used by permission.
†Excluding medical exposures.
‡Sum of external and internal exposures.
§Including background but excluding internal exposures.

The harmful effects of ionizing radiation are well known. New information regarding the stochastic effects continue to revise our philosophy on exposure limits for all. Table 9–16 summarizes the current exposure recommendations.

CONCLUSIONS

The welfare of the patient is of primary concern to all individuals in the medical field. The major aim is to offer maximum assistance to the patient with as little adverse effect as possible. As a result, the benefits versus the risks of procedures are constantly being weighed. The use of ionizing radiation for diagnostic purposes offers many benefits to the patient with minimal risks to individual health and to future generations. However, patients should always be exposed to as little radiation as possible.

Workers in radiation areas have a responsibility to themselves as well, and should not receive any unnecessary exposure. The guiding philosophy for dose limits for the occupationally exposed person is that exposure be kept "as low as reasonably achievable" to get the job done properly. Clearly, one can question what is reasonable, but this concept should stand any radiation worker in good stead.

All personnel in medical fields have a responsibility in the care of the patient and the minimizing of hazards. This is extremely important in diagnostic radiology and nuclear medicine, especially when the public is becoming more knowledgeable about and concerned with the hazards of radiation. The lay press has contributed to public concern and has reminded us of our responsibilities to our patients. Concern by the patient, coupled with the attention of the lay press, poses medicolegal problems for the medical profession. An increased amount of litigation has been directed against the medical profession, including radiology, particularly in the area of in utero exposure. Therefore, it is imperative from the standpoint of the patient's health, the health of personnel, the protection of future generations, and the avoidance of medicolegal problems that only the best and most judicious care be offered to the patient.

REFERENCES

1. Aboul-Khair SA, et al: Structural and functional development of the human foetal thyroid. *Clin Sci* 1966; 31:415.
2. American College of Radiology: *Medical Radiation: A Guide to Good Practice.* Chicago, ACR, 1985.
3. Atomic Energy Commission: *Medical Radionuclides: Radiation Dose Effects,* Proceedings of a Symposium, Oak Ridge Associated Universities, Oak Ridge, TN, 1969. Washington DC, US Government Printing Office, AEC Symposium Series 20, 1970.
4. Brent RL, Gorson RO: Radiation exposure in pregnancy, in Moseley RD (ed): *Current Problems in Radiology.* Chicago: Year Book Medical Publishers, 1972; 2(5):1–48.

5. Bureau of Radiological Health: *Gonadal Doses and Genetically Significant Dose from Diagnostic Radiology, U.S. 1964 and 1970.* US Department of Health, Education and Welfare, DHEW Publication (FDA) 76–8034. Washington DC, US Government Printing Office, 1976.

6. Court-Brown WM, et al: The incidence of leukemia following the exposure to diagnostic radiation in utero. *Br Med J* 1960; 2:1599.

7. Dalrymple GV, et al: *Medical Radiation Biology.* Philadelphia: WB Saunders, 1973.

8. Ford DD, et al: Fetal exposure to diagnostic x-rays in leukemia and other malignant disease in childhood. *J Natl Cancer Inst* 1959; 22:1093.

9. Gaulden ME: Possible effects of diagnostic x-rays on the human embryo and fetus. *J Arkansas Med Soc* 1974; 70:424.

10. Hammer-Jacobsen E: Therapeutic abortion on account of x-ray examination during pregnancy. *Dan Med Bull* 1959; 6:113.

11. Henry HF: *Fundamentals of Radiation Protection.* New York, John Wiley & Sons, 1969.

12. Kereiakes J, et al: Patient and personnel dose during radioisotope procedures, in *Medical Radiation Information for Litigation,* Proceedings of a Conference, Baylor University College of Medicine, Houston, November 21–22, 1968. Washington DC, US Government Printing Office, Publication No DMRE 69–3, 1969.

13. MacMahon B: Prenatal x-ray exposure and childhood cancer. *J Natl Cancer Inst* 1962; 28:1179–1191.

14. Margolis AR: Lessons of radiobiology for diagnostic radiology, Calwell Lecture, 1972. *Am J Roentgenol Radium Ther Nucl Med* 1973; 117:741.

15. Mettler FA: Diagnostic radiology: Uses and trends in the United States, 1964–1980. *Radiology* 1987; 162:263.

16. Mettler FA, Christie JH, Williams AG, et al: Population characteristics and absorbed dose to the population from nuclear medicine in the United States—1982. *Health Phys* 1982; 56:619.

17. Mole RH: Radiation effects in man; Current views and prospects. *Health Phys* 1971; 20:485.

18. Nader R: Wake up America; Unsafe x-rays! *Ladies Home Journal* May 1968, p 126.

19. National Council on Radiation Protection and Measurements: *Ionizing Radiation Exposure of the Population of the United States.* Washington DC, US Government Printing Office, Report No 93, 1987.

20. National Council on Radiation Protection and Measurements: *Medical Radiation Exposure of Pregnant and Potentially Pregnant Women.* Washington DC, US Government Printing Office, NCRP Report No 54, 1977.

21. National Council on Radiation Protection and Measurements: *Nuclear Medicine—Factors Influencing the Choice and Use of Radionuclides in Diagnosis and Therapy.* Washington DC, US Government Printing Office, NCRP Report No 70, 1982.

22. National Council on Radiation Protection and Measurements: *Protection in Nuclear Medicine and Ultrasound Diagnostic Procedures in Children.* Washington DC, US Government Printing Office, Report No 73, 1983.

23. National Council on Radiation Protection and Measurements: *Recommendations on Limits for Exposure to Ionizing Radiation.* Washington DC, US Government Printing Office, Report No 91, 1987.

24. National Council on Radiation Protection and Measurements: *Review of NCRP Radiation Dose Limit for Embryo and Fetus in Occupationally-Exposed Women.* Washington DC, US Government Printing Office, NCRP Report No 53, 1977.

25. Oliver R: 75 years of radiation protection. *Br J Radiol* 1973; 46:854.

26. Rosenstein M: *Organ Doses in Diagnostic Radiology.* Washington DC, US Government Printing Office, DHEW Publication (FDA) 76–8030, 1976.

27. Rugh R: *From Conception to Birth: The Drama of Life's Beginnings.* New York, Harper & Row, 1971.

28. Rugh R: Why radiobiology? *Radiology* 1964; 82:917.

29. Sagan LA: Human effects of low level radiation; A critique. *Proc Ninth Hannford Biology Symposium.* Atomic Energy Commission Symposium Series 17, 1969, pp 719–730.

30. Stein JJ: The carcinogenic hazards of ionizing radiation in diagnostic and therapeutic radiology. *Cancer* 1967; 17:278–287.

31. Sternglass EJ: Evidence for low level radiation effects on the human embryo and fetus. *Proc Ninth Hannford Biology Symposium,* Atomic Energy Commission Symposium Series 17, 1969, pp 651–660.

32. Stewart A, et al: A survey of childhood malignancies. *Br Med J* 1958; 1:1495.

33. Stewart A, Kneale GW: Radiation dose effects in relation to obstetric x-rays and childhood cancers. *Lancet* 1970; 1:1185.

34. Stewart A, et al: Malignant disease in childhood and diagnostic irradiation in utero. *Lancet* 1956; 2:447.

35. Stone RS: Common sense in radiation protection applied to clinical practice. *Am J Roentgenol Radium Ther Nucl Med* 1957; 78:993.

36. Stone RS: Concept of maximum permissible exposure; Carmen lecture. *Radiology* 1952; 58:639.

37. Warshofsky F: Warning—X-rays may be dangerous to your health! *Readers' Digest* August 1972; p 173.

Chapter 10_____

Clinical Radiobiology II: Therapeutic Radiology

Cancer is a leading cause of death in the United States today, second only to heart disease. Of every six deaths in the population, one is from cancer. The American Cancer Society estimated that there would be approximately 965,000 new cancer cases diagnosed in 1987. Of these, 483,000 people would die of this disease, 1,323 people a day, about one every 65 seconds. In the decade from 1970 to 1980 there were an estimated 3.5 million cancer deaths, 6.5 million new cancer cases, and 10 million persons under medical treatment for this disease.

Unfortunately, the word "cancer" still means inevitable death to many people; however, many people have been cured of this disease. The American Cancer Society estimates that today about 385,000 Americans or 4 out of 10 patients who were diagnosed with cancer in 1987 will be alive 5 years after diagnosis. This represents a significant improvement over the figures for even the 1960s, when only 1 out of 3 patients survived at least 5 years after treatment. The change from 1 to 3 to 4 in 10, although it appears small, means that 65,000 more people will survive their disease today than would have survived in the 1960s. Even more patients could be cured if their disease was detected and treated earlier. In 1987 alone, another 170,000 people will die who could have been saved by earlier diagnosis; another 20% or close to 6 out of 10 (rather than 4 out of 10) patients could be cured if they had sought treatment earlier. Today there are about 3 million Americans living who have been cured of cancer.

Ionizing radiation has long been used as a treatment for cancer, dating back to the discovery of x-rays and their lethal effects on tissues. For many years radiation therapy was regarded as a second treatment choice, to be used only when surgery was impossible or had failed. Today approximately 50% of all cancer patients receive radiation therapy for either curative or palliative (relief of symptom) purposes. Over the past two decades radiation therapy has made a great contribution to the improved 5-year survival of many cancer patients, e.g., those with Hodgkin's disease (6% survival rate in 1950; 80% in 1980) and seminoma (52% survival rate in 1950; 94% in 1970), while other types of cancer, e.g., lung cancer, have not reflected these improvements.

Radiation may be used alone in the treatment of certain malignant diseases, e.g., cervical carcinoma and early-stage Hodgkin's disease, or adjunctively (i.e., in combination) with another form of treatment such as surgery or chemotherapy, for diseases such as breast carcinoma. At present radiation therapy is a primary treatment modality and plays a significant and vital role in the management of patients with cancer.

GOAL OF RADIOTHERAPY

The goal of radiation therapy is to deliver a sufficiently high dose of radiation to sterilize the tumor cells with minimal damage to the surrounding normal tissues, with the ultimate result being complete eradication of the tumor with sufficient normal tissue remaining to ensure viability and function. Although this may appear at first glance to be an easily achievable goal, this is not always the case. It is a fact that treatment with radiation can cure tumors. As the dose of radiation is increased, more cells are killed, until, after a sufficiently high dose, all cells are killed and the tumor is eradicated. Usually this is achieved by giving high total doses in small daily fractions over a long period of time to only the localized tumor-bearing area. Thus, total doses of 50 to 70 Gy (or greater) can be delivered to this localized area without inducing any of the radiation syndromes or death. However, the interaction of radiation in matter, including cells, tissues, and organs, is a nonspecific, random process, with no specificity for tumor cells. The treatment area encompasses not only the tumor, but also surrounding normal tissues. In addition, radiation administered from sources outside the body is absorbed by normal tissues in its path to the tumor. Because the probability of radiation interacting with tumor cells is the same as the probability of interaction occurring in normal cells, damage occurs in normal tissues in the treatment area, as well as in the tumor.

As in the tumor, more cells are killed in the normal tissue as the dose is increased and the probability of damage occurring increases. However, all normal tissues have a limit as to the amount of radiation they can receive and still remain functional; this is defined as *radiation tolerance*. For this reason, the amount of radiation used to treat a specific malignant tumor is limited by the tolerance of the surrounding normal tissue, not by the tumor.

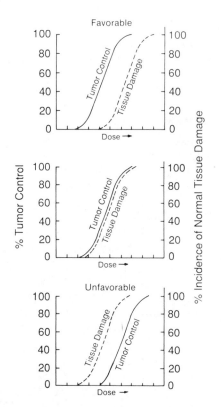

FIG 10–1.

Schematic of the relationship between tumor control and normal tissue damage as a function of dose of radiation. Clearly, the *top panel* is the ideal situation, where the dose for normal tissue damage is well above that for a high probability of tumor control. The least favorable situation would be where the dose for normal tissue damage is well below that for any probability of tumor control, as shown in the *bottom panel*. (Redrawn from P Rubin (ed): *Clinical Oncology: A Multidisciplinary Approach* New York, American Cancer Society, 1983.)

Although both the probability of tumor control and normal tissue damage are dose dependent, it is the difference in dose for the two situations that determines treatment outcome. This is termed the *therapeutic ratio*. Hypothetical dose-response relationships for the probability of tumor control and normal tissue damage are shown in Figure 10–1. Clearly, the ideal situation is when the dose-response curve for damage in the critical normal tissue sits well to the right (i.e., to higher total doses) than that for tumor control. In this case, a dose that gives a 90% probability of tumor cure may give less than 10% probability of normal tissue damage (Fig 10–1, top panel). Radiation therapy would be contraindicated when this situation is reversed, i.e., normal tissue damage occurs over a lower dose range than tumor control (Fig 10-1, lower panel). Unfortunately, in most cases, the two dose-response curves lie perilously close to each other (Fig 10–1, middle panel). Techniques such as treatment planning, dose fractionation schedules, and the LET of the radiation must be used, then, that take advantage of these relatively minor differences between normal and cancerous tissues.

The goal of radiotherapy, then, although dependent on cellular and tissue response in both the tumor and the normal tissue, is ultimately dependent on normal tissue response if complications are to be avoided (which may result in a cure no better than, and possibly worse than, the disease).

TUMOR RADIOBIOLOGY

General Tumor Characteristics

Malignant tumors, like normal tissues, are composed of a parenchymal compartment, i.e., the tumor cells and a stromal compartment consisting of normal blood vessels, lymphatic vessels and connective and nerve tissue. In general the parenchymal compartment consists of four subpopulations of tumor cells differing in viability and proliferative status:

- Group 1 - Well-oxygenated, viable, and actively proliferating (P-cells)
- Group 2 - Well-oxygenated, viable but not proliferating (Quiescent, Q-cells)
- Group 3 - Hypoxic but viable (also Quiescent, Q-cells)
- Group 4 - Anoxic and necrotic, i.e., not viable

Group 1.—This population, termed the *growth fraction* (GF), clearly is responsible for tumor growth. Observations of both experimental and animal tumors show a variation of 30% to 50% in the population of cells in this group. Clinically, though, this group may pose the least problem, since its actively dividing status coupled with its well-oxygenated state render these cells most sensitive to radiation, at least in relationship to the other groups.

Group 2.—Less clear is the role of this population in tumor growth and cure. Although the factors controlling the recruitment of Q-cells to P-cells is unknown, if recruited into cycle they obviously can contribute to tumor growth during, or even after, treatment causing a re-

TABLE 10–1.

Cell Cycle Times of the Cells of Solid Tumors and Their Normal Counterparts*

Normal Tissue	Cell Cycle Time (hours)	Tumors	Cell Cycle Time (hours)
Rat liver	21.5	Chemically induced hepatomas	14–16
Mouse skin	150	Epidermoid carcinomas	32
Mouse alveoli	64	Mammary tumors	33
Hamster cheek pouch epithelium	130–155	Chemically induced carcinomas	11
Rabbit epidermis	125–750	SPV-induced papillomas	21
Mouse stomach epithelium	28–55	Squamous cell carcinomas	8–12
Human cervical epithelium	100–600	Squamous cell carcinomas	15

*From Hall EJ (ed): *Radiobiology for the Radiobiologist.* Philadelphia, JB Lippincott, 1988, p 232. Used by permission.

currence. These cells could be one source that repopulates a tumor after treatment.

Group 3.—This population, which may constitute as much as 15% of the total viable cell population, may pose the biggest problem clinically. Although their hypoxic status makes these cells radioresistant (relative to the other cell populations in the tumor), they remain viable despite their poor oxygen supply. These cells may be another source that repopulates the tumor after therapy is completed.

Group 4.—These nonviable cells are of no consequence to tumor growth, nor to treatment outcome.

Tumor Growth

Tumor growth, measured in terms of doubling time (the time in which the tumor doubles in volume), is dependent on three factors:

1. The cell cycle time of the proliferating cells.
2. The growth fraction, i.e., the fraction of the total tumor cell population that is dividing.
3. The degree of cell loss from the tumor.

Cell cycle time.—In general, the cell cycle time of malignant cells is considerably shorter than that of their normal counterparts, as shown in Table 10–1. Measured in both animal and human tumors, this observation appears to imply a correspondingly short tumor volume dou-

servation appears to imply a correspondingly short tumor volume doubling time. Measured tumor doubling times, however, are much longer than expected based on these cycle times and range from 40 to 100 days. The median doubling time for human tumors is about 2 months, although there is a large variation among patients with the same tumor type. Although a small growth fraction may partially account for these apparently long doubling times, this factor alone cannot explain the discrepancy.

Growth fraction.—Critical to an understanding of tumor growth is the realization that not all the cells capable of proliferating in a tumor do so at the same time. The growth fraction is the ratio of *P*-cells (group 1 only) to *P* and *Q*-cells (made up of both groups 2 and 3 above). The growth fraction has been measured in some human tumors, and varies by a factor of 10 between rapidly dividing tumors (0.9 for lymphomas and embryonic tumors) and slowly dividing tumors (0.06 for adenocarcinomas). There appears to be a good correlation between the GF and volume doubling time—tumors with a high growth fraction have shorter doubling times.

Cell loss.—A third important factor is cell loss. Cells are lost from tumors in a number of ways, including metastases and cell death. Studies indicate a great variation in cell loss among different types of tumors (0% to 90%), with carcinomas exhibiting a greater cell loss than sarcomas. This observation may be a reflection of the growth characteristics of the normal tissue of origin: carcinomas arise from dividing, constantly renewing, epithelial cells; sarcomas from nonrenewing cell systems such as connective and soft tissue.

In human tumors the cell loss factor has been estimated to be between 50% and 80%, and appears to be higher in the faster growing tumors with high growth fractions. The cell loss factor may also account for the disparity between tumor cell cycle times (which, in general, are relatively short) and volume doubling times (which are long). Thus, although the dividing cells are doing so rapidly, a high degree of cell loss increases the time for the tumor to double in volume. In general, the pattern of tumor growth is determined by the rate of cell loss.

The rate of tumor growth, then, is a balance between three factors: cell cycle time, growth fraction, and cell loss.

Role of Oxygen in Tumor Growth

Malignant neoplasms are more complex tissues than originally believed. They appear to have some internal regulatory growth mechanisms. Unlike normal tissue, however, their unorganized growth pattern results in either an outgrowth of vascular supply or compression of vessels within the tumor. Both these situations produce the same result, a decrease of available oxygen to tumor cells.

A distinct architectural pattern consisting of a central region of necrosis surrounded by a rim of viable cells, termed a cancer cord, was observed in a human bronchial carcinoma by Thomlinson and Gray (Fig 10–2). Other tumors do not exhibit this characteristic pattern but contain many foci of necrosis. Further studies of the location of these distinctly different morphologic areas revealed them to be related to the size and growth of the tumor. Small tumors with a radius less than 100 μm did not exhibit a necrotic area, indicating sufficient vascular and, therefore, oxygen supply. As a tumor grew and its radius exceeded 160 μm, necrotic areas developed surrounded by a rim of viable cells between 100 and 180 μm in thickness. Continued tumor growth resulted in an increase in the size of the necrotic area, but the thickness of the rim of viable cells remained constant (Fig 10–3). Actual measurements of oxygen tension in these two areas demonstrated a much lower oxygen tension in the necrotic than in the viable tumor area,

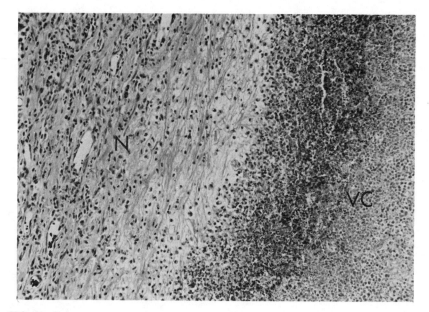

FIG 10–2.
Photomicrograph of a Walker 256 tumor grown in rats exhibiting a central region of necrosis *(N)* surrounded by a rim of viable cells *(VC)*. The cells visible in the necrotic area are inflammatory cells such as lymphocytes.

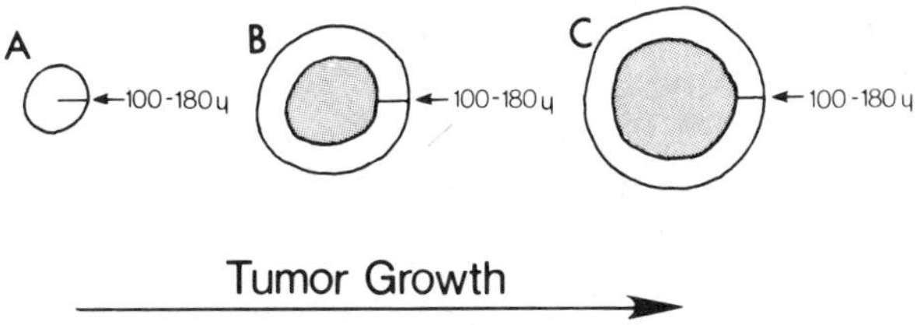

FIG 10–3.
Diagram of tumor growth illustrating constant width of rim of viable cells (100 to 180 μm) but increasing size of necrotic area as tumor increases in size.

implying either an insufficient vasculature or oxygen diffusion. Apparently, oxygen was not only a necessary requirement for life of the tumor cell, but also was a determining factor in its ability to proliferate. Indeed, calculation of the diffusion distance of oxygen in tissues by Thomlinson and Gray revealed a decreasing oxygen concentration with increasing distance from a vessel, approaching zero at approximately 150 to 200 μm. The close correlation of this calculation with the observed constant width of the rim of viable tumor cells (100 to 180 μm) supported the experimental supposition that oxygen was a critical factor in tumor growth.

In actuality, a clear-cut border does not exist between well and poorly oxygenated tumor areas; instead, there is a gradient of oxygen tension within a tumor, the highest appearing next to vessels and gradually decreasing with increasing distance from the vessel. Tumors can be considered as consisting of various compartments dependent on oxygen supply. Tumor cells greater than 180 μm from a vessel have no oxygen (are *anoxic*) and will not only be unable to proliferate but also will die, forming a necrotic area. Cells closest to a vessel are well oxygenated and may be actively dividing; these cells constitute the growth fraction. Between these extremes, a gradual decrease of oxygen tension produces increasing degrees of hypoxia; cells in this area, although not dividing, may be viable and capable of dividing. This hypoxic group of cells may make up 15% of the total number of viable cells.

The vasculature plays a vital role in both tumor growth and the ability of radiation to eradicate the tumor. Cells 180 μm from a blood vessel, (group 4 as described above) are nonviable and are not a problem in radiotherapy. Those cells closest to a vessel (group 1) also are not a major problem; they have a normal oxygen supply and are relatively sensitive to radiation. However, those cells that are not proliferating (group 2) or are hypoxic but viable (group 3) may pose the biggest problem, because they are relatively resistant to radiation compared with proliferating, well-oxygenated cells. These cells (groups 2 and 3) ultimately may be responsible for regrowth of the tumor.

The relationship of the populations of tumor cells to each other and to the tumor vasculature is shown in Figure 10–4.

RADIOSENSITIVITY AND RADIOCURABILITY

Tumors, like normal tissues, vary in their sensitivities to radiation; certain types of tumors are more sensitive than others. This is reflected in the total doses needed for cure for different tumors.

Table 10–2 gives a list of curative doses for different tumor types, showing that radiocurability varies by as much as a factor of 3. One interpretation of these data is that the tumor cells in breast cancers, for example, are three times more resistant to radiation than those in a seminoma, implying that the intrinsic radiosensitivity of tumor cells varies widely. However, using the parameter D_o, a standard measure of radiosensitivity, it has been shown that there is little variation in the D_o value for different human tumors that span this same range of clinical response. For example, the D_o for human melanoma cells cul-

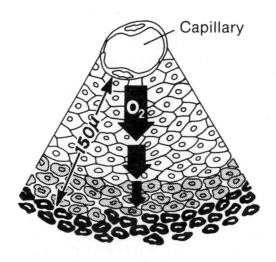

FIG 10–4.
Schematic of the relationship of the four populations of cells in the tumor to each other and the vasculature. Cells closest to the capillary are well-aerated *Q-* or *P*-cells, whereas the dark cells at the periphery (the farthest away from the capillary) are necrotic cells. The gray-shaded cells represent hypoxic but viable cells. Note that oxygen decreases with distance from the capillary (see text for further discussion). (Redrawn from Hall EJ: *Radiobiology for the Radiologist,* ed 3. Philadelphia, JB Lippincott, 1988. Used by permission.)

tured in vitro (a tumor which requires 80 Gy for cure) was 1.58 Gy, while the D_o for lymphomas (tumors that require only half that dose for cure) was similar, 1.21 Gy. What did correlate well with clinical

TABLE 10–2.
Curative Doses of Radiation for Different Tumor Types*

Dose Range (Gy)	Tumor
20–30	Seminoma
	Acute lymphocytic leukemia
30–40	Seminoma
	Wilms' tumor
	Neuroblastoma
40–45	Hodgkin's disease
	Lymphosarcoma
	Seminoma
	Histiocytic cell sarcoma
	Skin cancer (basal and squamous)
50–60	Lymph nodes, metastatic
	Squamous cell carcinoma, cervical cancer, and head and neck cancer
	Embryonal cancer
	Breast cancer, ovarian cancer
	Medulloblastoma
	Retinoblastoma
	Ewing's tumor
	Dysgerminomas
60–65	Larynx (<1 cm)
	Breast cancer
70–75	Oral cavity (<2 cm, 2–4 cm)
	Oro-naso-laryngo-pharyngeal cancer
	Bladder cancers
	Cervical cancer
	Uterine fundal cancer
	Ovarian cancer
	Lymph nodes, metastatic (1–3 cm)
	Lung cancer (<3 cm)
⩾80	Head and neck cancer (>4 cm)
	Breast cancer (>5 cm)
	Glioblastomas (gliomas)
	Osteogenic sarcomas (bone sarcomas)
	Melanomas
	Soft tissue sarcomas (>5 cm)
	Thyroid cancer
	Lymph nodes, metastatic (>6 cm)

*From Rubin P (ed): *Clinical Oncology—A Multidisciplinary Approach.* New York, American Cancer Society, 1983. Used by permission.

response, however, were those parameters that describe the initial part of the survival curve: α, n, and D_q. These observations strongly suggest that it is the initial part of the survival curve, not the distal portion, that correlates well with clinical response of human tumors. In other words, it is the repair capabilities of individual tumor cells that may vary the most and ultimately determine tumor response. It has been suggested that qualitative and/or quantitative differences in the repair of potentially lethal damage may account for this variability.

Recent advances in tissue culture techniques have allowed the response of tumors from individual patients to be assessed. In one study of seven histologic groups in which clinical response was known to vary from highly responsive to poorly responsive, the radiosensitivity measured by initial survival curve parameters corresponded well with clinical responsiveness. Such techniques are now being used to attempt to predict the response of individual patients to radiation therapy.

NORMAL TISSUE

The importance of preserving the integrity of normal tissue was recognized early in radiation therapy, leading to dose fractionation techniques. Many different fractionation and protraction schedules and total doses were used in these early years to treat malignant disease. In an attempt to correlate these various time-dose relationships with clinical results, Strandqvist reviewed 280 cases of carcinoma of the skin and lip followed for 5 years. Plotting total dose and overall treatment time on a double-log plot, he developed a series of lines, termed isoeffect curves, relating the treatment schedule to clinical results, including cure of the disease, occurrence of severe late complications (skin necrosis) and early minor complications, such as skin erythema and moist and dry desquamation (Fig 10–5). Strandqvist observed that some time-dose relationships, although curing the disease, also produced severe late complications while others resulted in no severe late damage but the tumor recurred or persisted (Fig 10–6). The result of this and other determinations of isoeffect curves was the establishment of treatment schedules that did not exceed the *tolerance* of various normal tissues but still afforded a high probability of tumor control.

Tolerance can be defined as the total dose at which additional radiation will significantly increase the probability of occurrence of severe normal tissue reactions. Tolerance is a clinical concept, accounting for inherent radio-sensitivity of the parenchyma and stroma, repair capabilities of both, preservation of functional integrity and the

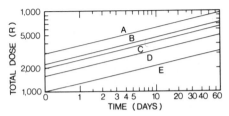

FIG 10–5.
Isoeffect curves drawn from Strandqvist's data relating various treatment schedules to clinical results: *A,* skin necrosis; *B,* cure of skin cancer; *C,* moist desquamation; *D,* dry desquamation; *E,* skin erythema. (From Strandqvist M: Studien über die kumulative Wirkung der Röntgenstrahlen bei Fraktionierung. *Acta Radiol [Suppl]* 1944; 55:1–300. Used by permission.)

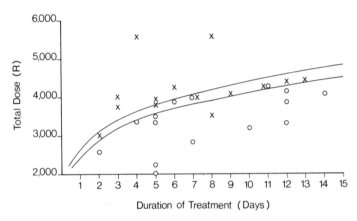

FIG 10–6.
Strandqvist's data plotted: the area between the two lines represents those time-dose relationships which gave a high probability of cure with a low probability of reactions. Cases above the line resulted in cures with late reactions, while the tumor persisted with no late reactions in those below the line. (From Strandqvist M: Studien über die kumulative Wirkung der Röntgenstrahlen bei Fraktionierung. *Acta Radiol [Suppl]* 1944; 55:1–300. Used by permission.)

importance of the organ to life. A better term than radiosensitivity in the clinical situation, tolerance indicates the variation in response of different organs to the same dose or range of doses. When tolerance is exceeded, the patient exhibits objective and subjective signs and symptoms of damage in the organ.

To better express tolerance, the concept of "tolerance dose" has been put forth. A modification of the $LD_{50/30}$ concept expressing lethality from total body radiation, the tolerance dose predicts the probability of complications occurring in different organs by various time-dose

TABLE 10–3.

Classification of Organ Tolerance Doses

Total Dose	Organs Exhibiting Complications
Low: 10–20 Gy	Gonads: ovaries and testes
	Developing organs, breasts, bone, and cartilage
	Bone marrow
	Lens
Moderate: 20–45 Gy	Stomach, intestine, colon (whole or major portion)
	Liver (35–45)
	Kidney (>25)
	Lung (>25)
	Heart (>45)
	Thyroid and pituitary glands
	Developing muscle
	Lymph nodes
High: 50–70 Gy	Epithelial structure, e.g., skin
	Oral cavity, esophagus, rectum, salivary glands, pancreas, bladder
	Mature bone and cartilage
	Organs of special sense, eye, ear
	CNS—brain and spinal cord
	Adrenals
Very high: >75 Gy	Ureters, vagina, urethra
	Mature breasts
	Muscle, blood, bile ducts

relationships. Because tolerance must be defined in terms of time and because survival from cancer is usually based on a time interval of 5 years, the tolerance dose is defined as the total dose delivered by a standard fractionation schedule that causes a minimum (5%) or maximum (50%) complication rate in 5 years. The tolerance dose therefore is expressed either as $TD_{5/5}$ (that dose which, when given to a population of patients, results in the minimum—5%—severe complication rate within 5 years posttreatment) or $TD_{50/5}$ (that dose which, when given to a population of patients, results in the maximum—50%—severe complication rate in 5 years).

Tolerance dose is a clinically practical concept, allowing the therapist to predict with some certainty the risk of inducing severe complications in patients treated using a specific time-dose relationship for a specific malignant disease. Most radiotherapists are unwilling to exceed the minimum of 5% complications, depending on the complication. For some normal tissues, even a 1% complication rate is considered unacceptable, e.g., myelopathy resulting from spinal cord irradiation. Tolerance doses of various organs classified as low, moderate, high, and very high irradiation are presented in Table 10–3. Table 10–4 lists the minimum and maximum tolerance doses and the type of injury that occurs for some selected vital organs whose destruction would result in death. The doses are based on standard fractionation schedules, i.e., 10 Gy/wk, 2 Gy/day, and 5 day/wk. Table 10–4 also shows that tolerance is clearly dependent on the volume of the organ irradiated; with increasing volume the total dose must be reduced if the acceptable complication rate is not to be exceeded.

Time-Dose Fractionation

Radiation therapy treatment schedules deliver a high total dose to the treatment area by dividing the dose into daily fractions administered over a period of time. That is, the dose is said to be fractionated and the time over which it is given is protracted. The total dose, the size of the fractions, the number of fractions and the time over which the treatment is given are determined by both the tumor and the tolerance of the surrounding normal tissue.

TABLE 10–4.

Class I Organs: Fatal/Severe Morbidity*

Organ	Injury	$TD_{5/5}$[†] (Gy)	$TD_{50/5}$[‡] (Gy)	Whole or Partial Organ (field size or length)
Bone marrow	Aplasia,	2.5	4.5	Whole
	pancytopenia	30	40	Segmental
Liver	Acute and chronic	25	40	Whole
	hepatitis	15	20	Whole (strip)
Stomach	Perforation, ulcer,	45	55	100 cm
	hemorrhage			
Intestine	Ulcer, perforation,	45	45	400 cm
	hemorrhage	50	65	100 cm
Brain	Infarction, necrosis	50	60	Whole
Heart	Pericarditis,	45	55	60%
	pancarditis	70	80	25%
Lung	Acute and chronic	30	35	100 cm
	pneumonitis	15	25	Whole
Kidney	Acute and chronic	15	20	Whole (strip)
	nephrosclerosis	20	25	Whole
Fetus	Death	2	4	Whole

*From Rubin P (ed): *Clinical Oncology—A Multidisciplinary Approach.* New York, American Cancer Society, 1983. Used by permission.

[†]$TD_{5/5}$ = Minimal tolerance dose. The dose to which a given population of patients is exposed under a standard set of treatment conditions resulting in no more than a 5% severe complication rate within 5 years after treatment.

[‡]$TD_{50/5}$ = The maximal tolerance dose is defined as the dose to which a given population of patients is exposed under a standard set of treatment conditions, resulting in a 50% severe complication rate within 5 years after treatment.

Dose fractionation techniques originated in 1927 with the observation that cells in the testis of a ram could be sterilized while producing little damage to the overlying skin of the scrotum if the total dose was divided into fractions rather than if given in a single exposure. The germinal cells of the testis were considered a suitable tumor model while the overlying scrotal skin represented a dose-limiting normal tissue, and this technique was applied to the treatment of cancer with radiation.

Biologically, fractionated doses are less efficient in causing cell death than are single doses; a higher total dose is necessary to produce the same degree of biologic damage when the dose is fractionated than when it is given as a single dose. Although fractionated doses would seem to favor tumor growth, years of experience have shown them to be more effective in controlling tumors, with a minimum of normal tissue damage, than large single doses.

We now know, 60 years after this original experiment, that the biologic effect on the tumor and normal tissue of fractionation is dependent on an interplay of four factors: repair, regeneration, redistribution, and reoxygenation. Termed the 4Rs of radiotherapy, these four factors are discussed below in increasing order of their probable importance to radiotherapy.

Redistribution*.—A dose of radiation has two effects on a dividing population of cells: (1) it causes a delay in the progression of cells in the cell cycle; and (2) the surviving population tends to be synchronized in resistant phases of the cell cycle (because the more sensitive [G2] cells were killed). In addition, there is a fivefold difference in survival after a dose of 2 Gy (the size of dose/per fraction used most often in radiotherapy), between the most resistant (late S) and the most sensitive (G2M) phases of the cell cycle (see Chapter 5). Thus, one would expect the net effect of fractionation to be a resistant population of cells. However, in most cases, this population rapidly becomes desynchronized and the net effect is sensitization of the surviving population (because the number of surviving cells redistributes into sensitive phases of the cell cycle).

Redistribution occurs in tumors and only in rapidly proliferating normal tissues such as skin, intestine, and esophagus. Theoretically, in a fractionated schedule, redistribution should result in increased cell kill in the tumor and acutely responding normal tissues, but should

---

*Redistribution is not the same as *recruitment* of noncycling (Q) cells into the cell cycle. Redistribution refers to the effect on cells already in cycle.

have no effect on late responding normal tissues (because the cells in these tissues divide slowly). This "R" then applies to the tumor, but only to acutely responding normal tissues. The overall effect of redistribution is difficult to measure, because by definition cycling cells are also proliferating cells, and thus any sensitizing effect of redistribution (in terms of reducing the dose) will be offset by the concomitant increase in cell numbers resulting from regeneration (which will necessitate a higher dose).

Reoxygenation.—It is clear that oxygen plays a critical role in cell killing by radiation (see Chapter 5). Cells that are hypoxic can be as much as three times more resistant to radiation than their well-oxygenated counterparts (i.e., it could take up to three times the dose to kill hypoxic cells than well-oxygenated cells). Thus, it is likely that oxygen also plays a role in the ability of radiation to cure tumors. This was clearly demonstrated in a mouse lymphosarcoma. When irradiated in vivo, a biphasic cell survival curve was obtained for this tumor (Fig 10–7). However, in vitro these cells gave an exponential survival curve.

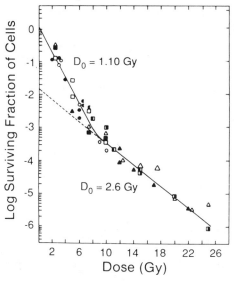

FIG 10–7.
Biphasic survival curve demonstrated for a lymphosarcoma grown and irradiated in vivo in a mouse. The first part of the survival curve has a steeper slope (D_o = 1.1 Gy) than the terminal portion of the curve, which has a shallower slope (D_o = 2.6 Gy), indicating that this tumor contains a proportion of hypoxic cells. (From Powers WE, Tolmach LJ: A multicomponent x-ray survival curve for mouse lymphosarcoma cells irradiated in vivo. *Nature* 1963; 197:710–711. Used by permission.)

The inflection in the in vivo survival curve was due to a proportion of hypoxic cells in the tumor (in this case, 1%). It is important to note that hypoxic cells determine the response only after high doses, well above those used in clinical radiotherapy. If human tumors do contain hypoxic cells (and there is no reason to assume that they do not), then radiotherapy would fail to cure any tumors, since even small tumors could contain as many as 10^9 cells which would not be cured by total doses of 70 Gy. However, fractionated regimens of radiation do work.

The most likely reason for the success of dose fractionation (if hypoxic cells are a problem in human tumors) is that the hypoxic cells reoxygenate during treatment. Fractionated radiotherapy would work in the following way:

A dose of radiation such as that used in conventional fractionation schedules (2 Gy/fraction) kills the well-oxygenated radiosensitive cells in a tumor. The oxygen status of the remaining hypoxic (radioresistant) cells then improves before the next dose fraction, rendering these cells now radiosensitive. This phenomenon, termed reoxygenation, probably plays a critical role in the ability of fractionated radiotherapy to cure at least some tumors. Since normal tissues are well oxygenated (relative to tumors), fractionating the dose over a protracted period of time should favor the killing of tumor cells that reoxygenate with little effect on critical normal tissues, thus improving the therapeutic ratio. This is the only one of the 4Rs that should selectively increase tumor cell kill.

Fractionated, protracted radiation does cure some human tumors, thus reoxygenation must be adequate between dose fractions. However, some tumors do fail conventional schedules. Although there may be alternative explanations as to why these tumors fail, it is likely that inadequate reoxygenation between dose fractions is at least partly responsible. Reoxygenation has been shown to vary considerably between different types of animal tumors.

One other consideration in reoxygenation is the magnitude of the oxygen effect after clinically relevant dose fractions of 2 Gy or less. Although difficult to measure, with new techniques it is now becoming obvious that the OER after low doses in the clinical range is less than 3. Thus, the influence of hypoxic cells may be less critical than originally believed, because they are less resistant after small doses in the clinical range. However, the OER even after small doses is still greater than 2; thus, it is likely that hypoxic cells and the failure to control them with conventional radiotherapy contributes at least partially to our inability to control at least some tumors with radiation. Ways of identifying hypoxic tumor cells in human tumors and minimizing their influence on treatment outcome have been a major area of radiobiology research and will be discussed in a later section.

Regeneration.—Cells in both normal tissues and tumors respond to the depopulation caused by a dose of radiation by regenerating, thereby repopulating both the tumor and the normal tissue. In normal tissues the time of onset of regeneration varies between tissues, depending on the cellular proliferation rate, because radiation induced cell death is linked to mitosis. Thus, tissues with high turnover rate (acutely responding), such as intestine and mucosa, will show compensatory proliferation during a fractionated course of radiotherapy, while those with more slowly proliferating cells (late responding), such as kidney and spinal cord, will exhibit little, if any, regenerative response during fractionated radiotherapy. Thus, protracting the overall treatment time will allow regeneration of surviving clonogenic cells and will be maximal in rapidly dividing tissue, but will be considerably less (if it occurs at all) in slowly proliferating tissues.

Regeneration, then, will occur in the tumor, and again only in acutely responding normal tissues. Although regeneration of surviving tumor cell clonogens is undesirable, regeneration and repopulation of the normal tissue is necessary if normal tissue tolerance is not to be exceeded.

Repair.—The fourth R, repair, refers strictly to cellular repair of radiation damage (SLD and PLD) (see Chapter 3), not to tissue repair by fibrosis. Repair may play the biggest role in the sparing effect of fractionation, because it occurs in both categories of normal tissues, acutely and late responding, as well as in tumors. In the past 5 years it has become obvious that acutely and late responding normal tissues differ in the total dose needed for isoeffect as the size of dose per fraction changes. This is shown in Figure 10–8, in which the total dose for isoeffect is plotted as a function of dose per fraction for damage in various normal tissues. Two distinct groups of curves can be seen: one group is relatively flat while the other increases steeply as the dose per fraction changes. The former represents acutely responding normal tissues, and the latter, late responding normal tissues. In the late responding group, the total dose for isoeffect increases more rapidly as the dose per fraction decreases. Put simply, these data suggest that small dose fractions will spare late responding normal tissues more than acutely responding normal tissues. Conversely, if the dose per fraction is increased, the total dose for isoeffect in late responding normal tissues will drop precipitously. It is this fact that was responsible for the unacceptable increase in complications when doses per fraction were doubled (from 2 to 4 Gy) in split-dose schedules.

The underlying biologic reason for the differences shown in Figure

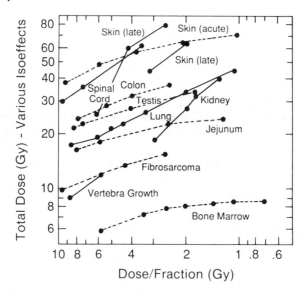

FIG 10–8.

Total dose for isoeffect for various normal tissues plotted as a function of dose per fraction. Two patterns can be seen. Some curves are very shallow *(dotted lines)*; they show little change in total isoeffect dose as a function of dose per fraction. Others are very steep *(solid lines)*, showing that the total dose for isoeffect changes rapidly as a function of dose per fraction. These represent acutely and late responding tissues, respectively. (From Thames HD, et al: Changes in early and late radiation responses with altered dose fractionation. Implications for dose survival relationships. *Int J Radiat Oncol Biol Phys* 1982; 8:219–226. Used by permission.)

10–8 is that the shape of the survival curves for the target cells of the two tissues may be different and that the cell survival curves of late effect tissues are "curvier" than acute effects tissues. This dissociation then is due to differences in repair capacity or shoulder shape of the underlying survival curves for the two categories of normal tissue. Thus, the same decrease in dose per fraction will cause a larger increase in the total dose for isoeffective tissue damage in the late effects tissues than in the acute effects tissues, as illustrated in Figure 10–9. In other words, the late effects tissues are more sensitive to changes in size of dose per fraction. Decreasing the dose per fraction should therefore increase the tolerance of late responding normal tissues (e.g., lung and spinal cord) with little change in the tolerance of acutely responding tissues such as the intestine.

In terms of the linear-quadratic relationship between dose and effect, the α/β ratio should be larger for acutely responding than for late responding normal tissues. α/β ratios determined from fractionation experiments for a number of normal tissues in mice and rats are given in Table 10–5. These experimental data suggest that this hypothesis is correct.

The impact of this finding on clinical radiotherapy is even more dramatic if it is assumed that tumors exhibit fractionation parameters similar to *acutely* responding, not *late* responding normal tissues, i.e., they have high α/β ratios. This is not a totally unreasonable assumption, since tumor response, like the response of acute effects tissues, is determined by depopulation of dividing cells. Although α/β ratios have

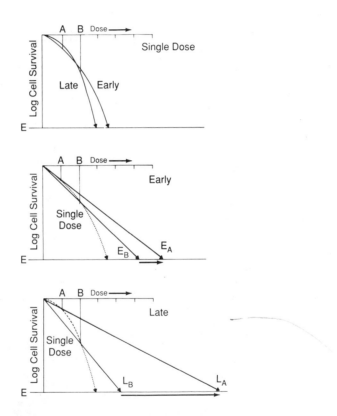

FIG 10–9.
Schematic of the effect of changing the size of dose per fraction on the total dose for isoeffect in an acutely responding and a late responding normal tissue. *Top panel* shows the single-dose survival curve for both an acutely responding tissue *(E)* and a late responding normal tissue *(L)*, showing that the late effects tissue has a "curvier" survival curve. The *middle and lower panels* show the effect of decreasing the dose per fraction from dose B to dose A on the total dose for isoeffect on an acutely and late effects tissue, respectively. The total dose for isoeffect changes very little, as the dose per fraction is reduced in an acute effects tissue, i.e., these tissues are insensitive to changing the dose per fraction *(middle panel)*. In contrast, the same reduction in dose per fraction in a late effects tissue results in the ability to give a much higher total dose for isoeffect. Late responding tissues, then, are more sensitive to changing the size of dose per fraction.

TABLE 10–5.

Estimates of α/β for Various Normal Tissues*

Tissue	α/β in Gy (95% confidence limits)
Acutely responding	
Skin	9.4 (6.1–14.3)
(desquamation)	11.7 (9.1–15.4)
	21.0 (16.2–27.8)
	10.5 (8.5–12.5)
Hair follicles	
(epilation)	
(anagen)	7.7 (7.4–8.0)*
(telogen)	5.5 (5.2–5.8)*
Lip mucosa	7.9 (1.8–25.8)
(desquamation)	
Jejunum	7.1 (6.8–7.5)
(clones)	
Colon	8.4 (8.3–8.5)
(clones)	
Testis	13.9 (13.4–14.3)
(clones)	
Spleen	8.9 (7.5–10.9)
(clones)	
Late responding	
Spinal cord	2.5 (−0.7–7.7)
(paralysis)	3.4 (2.7–4.3)
(cervical)	4.1 (2.2–6.5)
(lumbar)	5.2 (2.0–10.2)
Brain ($LD_{50/10\ mos}$)	2.1 (−1.1–14.4)
Eye (cataracts)	1.2 (0.6–2.1)
Kidney	
Rabbit	0.4 (−0.8–3.4)
Mouse	
(urination frequency)	1.6 (0.7–2.4)
(^{51}Cr-EDTA clearance)	4.1 (3.1–5.2)
Bladder	
(urination frequency)	7.2 (1.3–18.1)
(contraction)	7.8 (2.6–17.0)
Lung (LD_{50}/pneumonitis)	2.1 (0.2–5.2)
	2.5 (2.0–3.2)
	4.3 (3.8–4.9)
	3.0 (2.4–3.6)
	3.7 (3.2–4.3)
	3.7 (2.8–4.5)
Bowel	3.0–5.0 (−1.6–22.0)
(stricture/perforation)	
Total-body irradiation	5.1 (−1.5–15.0)
($LD_{50/1\ yr}$)	

*From Thames HD, Hendry JH: *Fractionation in Radiotherapy.* London, Taylor & Francis, 1987; pp 53–99. Used by permission.

been determined for many acute and late effects tissues and are consistently higher for the former, there are no values of α/β for human tumors. A review by Williams, Denekamp, and Fowler of experimental mouse tumors indicates, however, that α/β ratios for many tumors lie in the range of those for acute effects tissues and clearly outside the range of values for late effects. To the extent that these mouse tumor data are relevant to human tumors, decreasing the dose per fraction should not decrease the local tumor control.

The following summarizes the effects of the 4Rs in the two categories of normal tissues and, by inference, tumors:

1. Fraction size is the dominant factor in determining reactions in late responding normal tissue; overall treatment time has little effect.
2. *Both* fraction size and overall treatment time determine the response in acutely responding normal tissues and tumors.

Multiple Fractions Daily

An understanding of these differences in the fractionation responses of normal tissue and tumors has led to the implementation of fractionation schedules in clinical radiotherapy using more than one fraction a day. Termed Multiple Fraction Daily (MFD), these can be divided into two categories, which have quite different objectives.

Hyperfractionation.—The primary objective of this regimen is to spare late responding normal tissues by decreasing the size of dose per fraction. The overall treatment time is similar to that used in conventional schedules (6 to 8 weeks) but the number of fractions is doubled (at least) and the total dose is increased. Theoretically, this regimen should spare late responses (because the dose per fraction is reduced) while providing the same tumor control and acute reactions.

Accelerated fractionation.—The primary rationale here is to increase cell killing in the tumor by reducing the overall treatment time. The total dose remains the same as in a conventional schedule, as does the dose per fraction, but the treatment time is halved, because two fractions are given per day. Clinically it is difficult to complete such a treatment regimen without a break because acute reactions become dose limiting. Theoretically this regimen should increase tumor control (by reducing repopulation in rapidly proliferating tumors), but will have no effect on late responding normal tissues (because the dose per fraction remains the same).

In both schedules, the time between the fractions must be long enough to allow complete repair of sublethal damage.

Thames and co-workers recently reviewed data obtained from clinical trials using these two MFD regimens. Most of the data were obtained from the treatment of head and neck cancers. In general, it was found that MFD treatments, whether with accelerated or hyperfractionation, were associated with increased severity of acute effects (as predicted). Late effects were generally equivalent or reduced in hyperfractionated schedules (as predicted). This is one example in which radiobiological data have been used to change radiotherapy practice in a prospective manner.

Isoeffect Formulae

The fractionation (time-dose) parameters that influence the tolerance of normal tissues are total dose, overall treatment time, size of dose per fraction, and spacing of dose fractions.

The different time-dose relationships in radiotherapy used to treat various malignant diseases are usually expressed as total dose and number of days over which treatment is given, e.g., 50 Gy in 5 weeks and 60 Gy in 6 weeks. Inherent in these figures is the understanding that these schedules do not exceed the tolerance of normal tissues surrounding the tumor. Because treatment schedules for the same disease may vary among radiotherapists, and because clinicians may choose to change fractionation schedules, several formulae have been proposed that will predict equivalent normal tissue reactions for different treatment schedules or for a change in treatment schedule. The most notable of these are the NSD formula and the α/β ratio.

Nominal standard dose (NSD).—This model was important in that it separated the number of fractions (N) from overall treatment time (T) in determining isoeffect dose by the relation:

$$\text{Total Dose} = \text{NSD}^{T^{0.11}N^{0.24}}$$

It was one of the simplest and most widely used formulae and has been much discussed. However, the NSD failed clinically because it did not predict damage in late responding normal tissues. In addition, it overestimated isoeffect doses for both very small and very large numbers of fractions (i.e., the tissue would be overdosed).

The primary reasons for its failure lie in two assumptions of the model:

1. It assumed that the capacity to repair sublethal damage is the same for *all* normal and malignant cells.
2. It assumed that the effect of fractionation is the same in *all* normal tissues.

Clearly, neither of these assumptions applies, and, in fact, the NSD is now known to be clearly inappropriate for predicting late effects.

α/β model.—This model is an improvement over the NSD in that it recognizes the differences between the fractionation responses of acute and late responding normal tissues and does predict the differential effect of changing the size of dose per fraction on the effects in these two categories of normal tissues.

Clearly, however, none of these models should be used as anything other than a guideline for making changes in clinical practice. Any regimen predicted by any model must be clinically tested to insure its safety.

CHEMICAL MODIFIERS IN RADIOTHERAPY*

The basic rationale for the use of any modifier in clinical radiotherapy is to increase the dose differential for tumor control and normal tissue complications, i.e., improve the therapeutic ratio. This can be accomplished either by sensitizing the tumor or protecting the normal tissue. The optimum situation is where the modifier acts selectively, changing the response of only the tumor or normal tissue, but not both.

Radiosensitizers

Radiosensitizers are drugs which increase the lethal effects of radiation when given in conjunction with it. Obviously, for use in clinical radiotherapy, these drugs must increase the sensitivity of only tumors to radiation. The basic rationale for the use of radiosensitizers is shown in Figure 10–10. These drugs improve the therapeutic ratio by moving the tumor control curve to the left (to lower doses) without affecting the complication curve for the critical normal tissue. Although many drugs have been described which are radiosensitizers, only two classes

---

*The discussion of chemotherapeutic agents is beyond the scope of the chapter. The interested reader is referred to *Radiobiology for the Radiologist*, by Eric J. Hall, for a discussion of chemotherapy from the radiobiologist's and radiotherapist's perspective (see References).

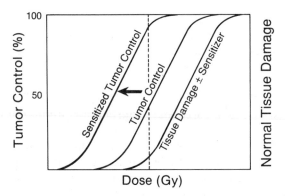

FIG 10–10.
Schematic of the rationale for using sensitizers in radiotherapy. The sensitizer shifts the tumor control curve to lower radiation doses while not affecting the normal tissue complication curve; therefore, the therapeutic ratio would increase because the sensitizer would affect only the tumor and not the normal tissue. (Adapted from Hall EJ: *Radiobiology for the Radiologist,* ed 3. Philadelphia, JB Lippincott Co, 1988.)

of drugs fit the criteria of providing a differential between the tumor and normal tissue: (1) hypoxic cell sensitizers, and (2) halogenated pyrimidines.

Hypoxic cell sensitizers.—Two relevant questions must be asked concerning the use of these compounds in the clinic: (1) Do human tumors contain hypoxic cells? and (2) Are they important in the ability of radiation to cure tumors? Although the evidence for hypoxic cells in human tumors is only circumstantial (Table 10–6), based on this and the animal data, efforts to sensitize hypoxic cells in human tumors could be productive. Based on the laboratory studies, the radiosensitizer misonizadole (MISO) was introduced into a large number of clinical trials in many different types of tumors. Unfortunately, the results have been disappointing. Only one trial showed a clear advantage to using MISO, and only when the patients were carefully divided into subgroups based on disease (cancer of the pharynx) and hemoglobin (Hb) level. Patients with high Hb levels given MISO showed significantly better tumor control compared with those with significantly lower Hb levels also given MISO, 61% vs. 28% tumor control at 3 years, respectively. The finding that Hb level was important in tumor control added significantly to the suspected role of hypoxic cells in ultimate tumor control.

Although a dose-limiting toxicity was not identified for MISO in the laboratory, a dose-limiting toxicity—peripheral neuropathy—was found when the drug was entered into clinical trials. The effect of this toxicity has been to limit the dose of drug that can be given in a

TABLE 10–6.

Circumstantial Evidence for Existence of Radiobiologically Hypoxic Cells in Human Tumors*

1. Histology showing necrosis at distances from capillaries consistent with oxygen depletion.
2. Polarographic measurements of pO_2 in tumors.
3. Increased mean intercapillary distance as measured colposcopically in carcinoma of cervix.
4. Increased acidity in venous blood from tumors (implying anaerobic respiration).
5. Improved local control rates in hyperbaric oxygen compared with air when large radiation dose fractions are used.
6. Enhancement of tumor response to large radiation dose fractions by chemical sensitizers of hypoxic cells.

*From Withers HR, Peters LJ: Biological aspects of radiation therapy, in Fletcher GH (ed): *Textbook of Radiotherapy*, Philadelphia, Lea & Febiger, 1980, pp 103–180. Used by permission.

---

fractionated regimen. Thus, the poor clinical results may be mostly due to the inability to administer adequate doses of the drug.

For this reason, new drugs were sought in the laboratory that were less toxic. Although the reason for such laboratory studies may seem unclear, (after all, laboratory studies with MISO did not identify its dose-limiting toxicity) the studies to define new less toxic sensitizers were beautiful in their logic. It was found that a minute change in the chemical structure of the drug resulted in other drugs that had similar sensitizing properties but with less toxicity. Two of this generation of compounds, SR2508 and RO03-8799, have been introduced into clinical trials and have been shown to be at least five times better than misonidazole. Based on these data, then, the future for selectively sensitizing hypoxic tumor cells may be promising.

Halogenated pyrimidine.—As discussed in Chapter 5, the halogenated pyrimidines IUdR and Brd Udr are structurally similar to thymidine such that, if present at the time of cell division, they will be incorporated into the DNA in place of thymidine, weakening the DNA chain and rendering that cell more sensitive to radiation. The rationale for the use of these drugs in clinical radiotherapy is that some tumor cells may cycle faster than the cells in the surrounding critical normal tissues. Clearly, these compounds should not be used if the tumor is surrounded by actively proliferating normal tissues (e.g., skin and intestine). Unfortunately, this was not appreciated in 1978 when these compounds were first tested clinically in head and neck cancers.

Although the tumor response was encouraging, normal tissue damage was unacceptable. Obviously these drugs fell out of favor until quite recently when the National Institutes of Health began a clinical trial using more appropriate tumor sites. These clinical data are not yet available for analysis, but this appears to be another promising avenue for improving the therapeutic ratio. Of particular benefit may be the use of these drugs with implant radiotherapy, since it has been found that the sensitizing effect of both IUdR and Brd Urd is the same with low dose rates as with the high dose rates used in conventional fractionation schedules. The advantage here is that the concentration of the halogenated pyrimidine required for sensitization can be more easily maintained during the week or so required for implant therapy than for the 6 weeks of conventional treatment.

Radioprotectors

The opposite side of the sensitization coin as an approach to improving the therapeutic ratio is selective protection of critical dose-limiting normal tissues. Schematically shown in Figure 10–11, the aim of these drugs is to shift the normal tissue curve to higher doses (to the right) without affecting the tumor cure curve. Drugs which afforded good protection against radiation damage were found as early as 1948, but their use in humans was, and still is, limited by their toxicity. The Walter Reed Army Hospital has synthesized and tested over 2,000 of

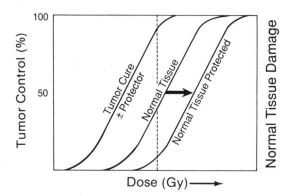

FIG 10–11.
The rationale for the use of radioprotectors in clinical radiotherapy. Ideally, radioprotectors should shift the curve for normal tissue responses to higher total doses, while having no effect on the tumor. Thus, a higher therapeutic ratio is achieved by changing the dose range over which normal tissue damage occurs. (Adapted from Hall EJ: *Radiobiology for the Radiologist,* ed 3. Philadelphia, JB Lippincott Co, 1988.)

these compounds, but only one of these, WR-2721, has made its way to the clinic.

The central issues in the use of WR-2721 in the clinic are: (1) its toxicity, (2) its ability to selectively protect normal tissues, and (3) its protective effect after small, clinically relevant dose fractions.

It is clear that the major toxicity of this drug in humans, hypotension, limits the dose that can be given to that which may be inadequate for maximum protection. Data are not yet available which answer this question.

Protection factors* for a variety of normal tissues are given in Table 10–7, showing that protection varies widely among the normal tissues tested. Although the reasons for this variation are not totally known, it is clear that tissue oxygenation is critical and that tissues with intermediate oxygen levels are better protected than either well-aerated or very poorly oxygenated ones. In addition, the values in Table 10–7 were obtained using large single doses of radiation, and therefore are applicable to only two clinical situations: intraoperative radiotherapy and total body irradiation. Since most treatment regimens use fraction-

TABLE 10–7.

Summary of Normal Tissue Responsiveness to Protection by WR2721*

Tissue	Protection Factor
Bone marrow	2.4–3
Immune system	1.8–3.4
Skin	2–2.4
Small intestine	1.8–2
Colon	1.8
Lung	1.2–1.8
Esophagus	1.4
Kidney	1.5
Liver	2.7
Salivary gland	2.0
Oral mucosa	>>1
Testes	2.1

*From Yuhas JM, Spellman JM, Culo F: The role of WR2721 in radiotherapy and/or chemotherapy, in Brady L (ed): *Radiation Sensitizers*. New York, Masson, 1980, pp 303–308. Used by permission.

*Protection factor $= \dfrac{\text{Dose with protector}}{\text{Dose without protector}}$ for same biological effect.

ated doses on the order of 2 Gy, the usefulness of WR-2721 depends on its ability to protect after small dose fractions. Experimental data, although limited, show that protection does decrease with reduction in dose. However, in most tissues, the protection factor even after low doses ranges from 1.1 to 1.2, indicating that total doses could be escalated by 10% to 20% without increasing the complication rate. More importantly, a 10% to 20% increase in total radiation dose could significantly improve tumor control, if tumors are not protected by these drugs.

This brings us to the third critical issue in the clinical use of any radioprotector: Does it protect tumors? Experimental data, although not extensive, indicate that they probably do not.

In summary, the use of radioprotectors in the clinic is still problematic, with many key issues regarding its use unresolved.

NEW RADIATION MODALITIES

Neutrons

Neutrons were used in clinical radiotherapy as early as the 1940s. However, because the difference in the shapes of cell survival curves for neutrons and x-rays was not known, a large number of patients were overdosed and exhibited unacceptable normal tissue damage. With the important knowledge that cell survival curves for neutrons were straighter than those for x-rays (i.e., neutron survival curves had little shoulder) an adjustment in total dose was made so that normal tissue reactions were not unacceptable, and neutron therapy again became accepted.

Neutrons have two advantages biologically over x-rays in clinical radiotherapy: (1) cell killing is less dependent on oxygen, and (2) neutrons reduce the variability in initial shoulder size and shape. However, neutrons will only be useful clinically if they show a larger RBE for tumors than for normal tissues at the same dose/fraction. It is well known (see Chapter 5) that the RBE after doses per fraction in the clinical range is higher for late responding normal tissues than for acutely responding normal tissues (see Fig 10–12). What this means is that the late responding normal tissues will be dose limiting for neutrons. Although a great deal of experimental data are available on the RBEs for most normal tissues, tumor data are sparse. Those few data available from murine tumors also are plotted in Figure 10–13, as RBE as a function of dose/fraction. These data show that the RBE for tumors is also dose dependent and falls within the limits of the two critical normal tissues at equivalent doses, as shown in Figure 10–13. The data

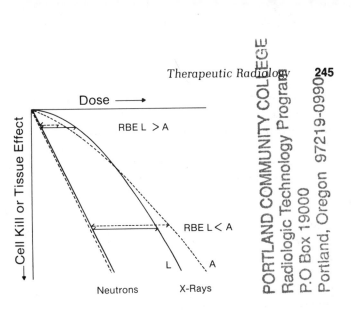

FIG 10–12.
Hypothetical survival curve for the target cells of an acute effects *(dotted line, A)* and a late effects *(solid line, L)* normal tissue to x-rays or neutrons. The late effects cells have a "curvier" survival curve than the acute effects cells, thus the RBE will be higher for late effects tissues than for acute effects tissues after low doses. (From Travis EL, Peters LJ, Barkley T: *Lung Cancer, Current Status and Prospects for the Future.* University of Texas Press, Austin, Texas, 1986. Used by permission.)

of Battermann and co-workers for human tumors are perhaps more relevant. These authors found that the neutron RBE for growth delay of human pulmonary metastases was related to the volume-doubling time of the tumors; that is, the longer the doubling time, the higher the RBE. These data imply that neutrons would be most useful in slowly growing tumors. The experimental findings are supported by clinical data indicating that neutrons are superior in treating prostate cancer and soft tissues sarcomas, both slowly growing tumors.

In general, although the biologic rationale for using neutrons is compelling, the clinical data are less so. True, the clinical trials, like most clinical trials, were hampered in some way—patient selection and small numbers—just two of the weak points—but with the exception of prostate cancer, salivary gland tumors, soft tissue sarcomas, and perhaps some head and neck tumors, to date neutrons have shown little, if any, advantage over x-rays.

Neutrons? Hyperfractionation?—It is interesting to compare neutrons with the new MFD schedules discussed earlier in terms of patient selection. Tumor volume doubling times could be useful here. For example, slowly growing tumors would be best treated with neutrons. Tumors with doubling times between 10 and 100 days would be best treated with a hyperfractionated schedule. If the doubling time is less than 10 days, however, a treatment schedule that shortens the overall treatment time, such as accelerated fractionation, should be employed. Because little is known about the doubling time of human tumors, other clinical information must be obtained from each patient that will best match patient to treatment alternative. The Battermann study of human lung metastases showed a correlation between tumor volume-doubling time and differentiation; i.e., well-differentiated tumors had doubling times of more than 100 days, whereas the doubling time of poorly differentiated tumors was shorter than ten days. Based on these data, then, well-differentiated tumors would be best treated with neutrons, moderately differentiated ones with hyperfractionation, and poorly differentiated tumors with an accelerated fractionation schedule. To the extent that these findings in human lung metastases apply to other human tumors, routine pathologic examinations could be useful in matching patients to treatment regimens.

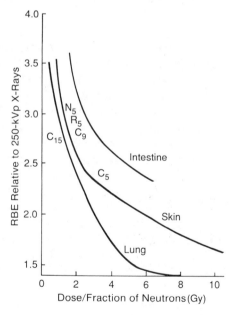

FIG 10–13.
RBE for three normal tissues and some experimental tumors, as a function of dose per fraction. It is clear that the RBE increases as the dose per fraction is decreased, and that the values for the few experimental tumors measured all lie within the range of the normal tissues tested (kVp = kilovolts peak). (From Field SB: An historical survey of radiobiology in radiotherapy with fast neutrons. *Curr Top Radiat Res Q* 1976; 11:1–86. Used by permission.)

Protons

The appeal of proton use in clinical radiotherapy is not biologic (their radiobiologic properties, RBE and OER, are indistinguishable from x-rays), but physical. Because of their dose distribution—a sparsely ionizing path that ends abruptly with a very high LET peak (called the *Bragg peak*), after which the dose quickly falls off to zero—it is possible to confine the dose to the tumor volume with minimal dose to surrounding normal tissues. Protons offer an advantage over conventional modalities only in treatment situations in which a sharp dose cutoff is necessary, such as for tumors located near the spinal cord.

Heavy Ions

The use of heavy ions in clinical radiotherapy is based on radio-biologic premises: in the Bragg peak, cell killing is independent of oxygen; the OER approaches unity, and the RBE in this same region is very high. The Bragg peak of these ions can be placed deep inside the body by increasing the energy of the particles, and can be used to treat deep-seated tumors.

The only unit in the world that produces these heavy ion beams for clinical application is at the University of California at Berkeley. Clinical trials have been ongoing using this machine, but the results have been unremarkable. As with the neutron trials, patient selection is not optimal and tumor types vary widely. Thus, any advantage could be swamped by inability to choose patients who might benefit the most from this modality.

Pions

Like protons, the major advantage of pions is their depth dose pattern, although there are biologic advantages too, e.g., high RBE and decreased OER in the Bragg peak. Clinical trials are ongoing in two facilities, the TRIUMF in Vancouver, British Columbia, and another in Cern, Switzerland. These trials are not completed, so it is not known whether pions will improve tumor control.

NEW TREATMENT TECHNIQUES

Two new treatment techniques that depart from the convention of fractionation and localized irradiation are being used in selected diseases. These are intraoperative radiotherapy (IORT) and total body irradiation (TBI).

Intraoperative Radiotherapy

As the terminology implies, this technique delivers radiation directly to a deep-seated tumor-bearing area during surgery. This technique would be most useful in diseases where the volume of normal tissue to be irradiated is prohibitive to the delivery of a curative dose to the tumor. Cancers located in the abdomen are prime candidates, and, in fact, IORT is being used clinically for tumors in this site. A large single dose, on the order of 20 Gy, can be given to the tumor-bearing area with the aim of eradicating any residual disease while the intestines are physically moved out of the field. Because any remaining hypoxic cells would dominate the tumor response after such large single doses, chemical sensitizers or heat used in conjunction with IORT could improve the results.

Randomized clinical trials have been conducted in selected patients with abdominal tumors. A significant improvement in local control, 20% to 30%, was found after resection of pancreatic tumors, retroperitoneal sarcomas, and gastric tumors. Survival also was improved by 10% to 20%. In a nonrandomized clinical trial of advanced colorectal tumors, survival was improved by 30% to 40%.

Although this technique will be useful in only selected diseases, if it increases tumor control for such cancers as pancreatic cancer, for which results are uniformly dismal (it would be a welcome addition to the radiotherapy armamentarium).

Total Body Irradiation

Conventional treatments deliver high doses safely by irradiating only a localized area of the body. Total body irradiation (TBI) departs from this convention and thus is useful for a few selected diseases. TBI is most often used as a conditioning regimen in preparation for bone marrow transplantation in some leukemias. Clearly, in this situation, the bone marrow is the tumor and not the dose-limiting normal tissue. Thus, doses higher than those which cause death from bone marrow depletion can be given (because the patient's marrow will be replaced via transplantation) and must be given if the tumor is to be controlled. (The $LD_{50/30}$ dose for humans, 3.5 Gy, will not cure any cancer.) The primary dose-limiting tissue in this treatment setting is lung. If leukemic cells respond like normal bone marrow to radiation, either low

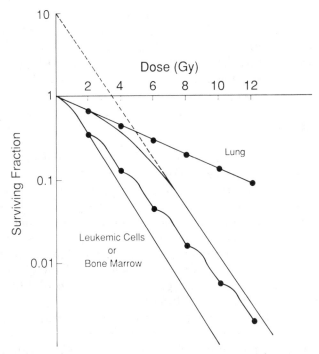

FIG 10–14.
Schematic of the rationale for using low dose rate or fractionated radiation when total-body irradiation is used as a preparative regimen for bone marrow transplantation. The target cells are the leukemic cells, whereas the lung is the critical dose-limiting normal tissue. Because of the difference in the shapes of the two survival curves for the target cells (leukemic cells and bone marrow having a very small shoulder, lung having a large shoulder), reducing the dose per fraction or using low-dose-rate irradiation should spare the lung more than the leukemic cells. (From Peters LJ: Discussion: The radiobiologic basis of TBI. *Int J Radiat Oncol Biol Phys* 1980; 6:785–787. Used by permission.)

dose rates or fractionated doses should spare the lung but not the leukemic cells because of the differences in the survival curves for lung and bone marrow, a late and acutely responding normal tissue, respectively (Fig 10–14).

In most centers, TBI is now given in a fractionated schedule, but controversy exists over the optimum dose rate. Clearly, some of this discussion is academic, since the dose rate is dictated by the need for longer treatment distances in order to irradiate the whole body. Experimental data suggest there is no dose rate effect at fraction sizes of less than 2.0 Gy. Thus, conventional dose rates (>1 Gy/min) offer the same therapeutic ratio as dose rates as low as 0.025 Gy/min given as fractionated doses or in a continuous schedule.

TBI is rarely (if ever) used alone but is most likely combined with one or more cytoreductive chemotherapy agents, many of which on their own are cytotoxic to the lung. Thus, the mechanism of lung damage in such schedules is hotly debated with as many investigators blaming the drugs as the radiation.

HYPERTHERMIA

It was reported as long as 100 years ago that cancers sometimes regressed in patients with fevers. However, only after logical laboratory experiments were performed in the last 20 years has the use of heat gained acceptance as a treatment for cancer. These experimental data have been augmented by preliminary clinical results which showed that significant tumor control could be achieved with heat alone or even better, with heat combined with x-rays. Thus, the current use of heat in cancer therapy (hyperthermia) has a sound biologic basis and is designed to exploit the known properties of heat cell killing which differ in many ways from cell killing by x-rays.

As with any other treatment, heat must provide a differential effect on the tumor and normal tissue to be useful in cancer therapy. The reasons why heat might provide a favorable therapeutic ratio in combination with x-rays are:

1. S-phase cells, which are resistant to radiation, are sensitive to heat.
2. Cell killing by heat is independent of oxygen, i.e., well-oxygenated and hypoxic cells are equally sensitive.
3. Heat inhibits the repair of SLD and PLD (an advantage to tumor control but a disadvantage to normal tissue damage).
4. Heat kills cells at low pH more readily than at normal pH. Thus, a given dose should kill more tumor cells than cells in the normal tissues.
5. Heat kills nutritionally deprived cells, a condition that favors tumor cell kill.
6. Heat preferentially damages tumor vasculature, again a factor in favor of tumor cell kill.
7. A poor blood supply, often associated with tumors, increases heat deposition.
8. Heat inhibits repair of DNA damage (which is favorable to tumor control, but a disadvantage to normal tissue damage).

As can be seen, there are significant differences in the ways in which heat and radiation kill cells such that a combination of the two modalities would be expected to improve the therapeutic ratio.

One important difference between the effect of radiation and heat on cells is that cells express their damage within hours after heating, i.e., cell death is not related to division as it is with radiation. This implies that the mechanism of cell killing by heat differs from that by radiation and that heat damage is unrelated to damage in DNA. Probable mechanisms for cell killing by heat are damage to the cell membrane and inactivation of proteins.

It is clear then that heat increases the damage to both tumors and normal tissues when used in conjunction with x-rays. Defined as the thermal enhancement ratio (TER), the TER can be expressed as:

$$\text{TER} = \frac{\text{Radiation dose without heat}}{\text{Radiation dose with heat}} \text{ for the same biological endpoint}$$

Because no consistent differences have been observed between the sensitivity of tumor cells compared with normal tissue cells to killing by heat, the question is whether heat improves the therapeutic ratio over x-rays alone. When combined with lower doses of x-rays, does it give higher tumor control for the same normal tissue damage than using higher doses of x-rays alone? Is there a therapeutic gain? If not, then it provides no advantage over higher doses of x-rays alone. Although the answer to this question is unclear, several clinical studies suggest that heat when combined with x-rays has the potential for improving tumor control.

Like all other modalities the use of heat in the clinic is not without its problems. Two problems currently limit the use of hyperthermia:

1. Engineering and physics—the ability to deliver and measure the heat dose in deep-seated tumors.
2. Thermotolerance—fractionated doses of heat or prolonged heating at temperatures of 40°C or less reduce cell killing to a subsequent dose, and the tissue becomes "tolerant" to another heat dose.

For the latter reason, and to take advantage of the complementary effects of the two modalities, heat might be added to one daily fraction of radiation on one of the days of each week of each treatment.

REFERENCES

1. Adams GE: Chemical radiosensitization of hypoxic cells. *Br Med Bull* 1973; 29:48–53.
2. Adams GE, et al: Electron affinic radiosensitization. *Int J Radiat Biol* 1969; 19:575.
3. American Cancer Society: *Cancer Facts and Figures.* New York, 1987.
4. Arcangeli G, Cevidalli A, Nervi C, et al: Tumor control and therapeutic gain with different schedules of combined radiotherapy and local external hyperthermia in human cancer. *Int J Radiat Oncol Biol Phys* 1983; 9:1125–1134.
5. Bagshaw MA, Doggett RL, Smith KC: Intra-arterial 5 bromodeoxy-uridine in x-ray therapy. *Am J Roentgenol* 1967; 99:889–894.
6. Battermann JJ, Breur K, Hart GAM, et al: Observations on pulmonary metastasis in patients after single doses and multiple fractions of fast neutrons and cobalt 60 γ-rays. *Eur J Cancer* 1981; 17:539–548.
7. Blakely EA, Edington MS (eds): Heavy charged particles in research and medicine. *Radiat Res* [Suppl] November 1985; 104:S1–S334.
8. Broerse JJ, Barendsen GW: Relative biological effectiveness of fast neutrons for effects on normal tissues. *Curr Top Radiat Res Q* 1973; 8:305–350.
9. Brown JM, Goffinet DR, Cleaver JE, et al: Preferential radiosensitization of mouse sarcoma relative to normal skin by chronic intra-aterial infusion of halogenated pyrimidine analogs. *J Natl Cancer Inst* 1971; 47:75–89.
10. Catterall M: Results of neutron therapy, differences, correlations, and improvements. *Int J Radiat Oncol Biol Phys* 1982; 8:2141–2144.
11. Dewey WC, Hopwood LE, Sapareto LA, et al: Cellular responses to combinations of hyperthermia and radiation. *Radiology* 1977; 123:463–474.
12. Ellis F: Dose, time, and fractionation, a clinical hypothesis. *Clin Radiol* 1969; 20:1–7.
13. Ellis F: Dose, time, and fractionation in radiotherapy, in Ebert M, Howard A (eds): *Current Topics in Radiation Research.* Amsterdam, North Holland Publishing Co, 1968, pp 359–397.
14. Ellis F: Nominal standard dose and the ret. *Br J Radiol* 1971; 44:101–108.
15. Field SB: An historical survey of radiobiology in radiotherapy with fast neutrons. *Curr Top Radiat Res Q* 1976; 11:1–86.
16. Field SB, Hornsey S: RBE values for cyclotron neutrons for effects on normal tissues and tumors as a function of dose and dose fractionation. *Eur J Cancer* 1971; 7:151–169.
17. Fowler JF: Dose response curves for organ function and cell survival. *Br J Radiol* 1983; 56:497–500.
18. Fowler JF: Forty years of radiobiology: Its impact on radiotherapy. *Phys Med Biol* 1984; 29:97–113.
19. Fowler JF: LaRonde-Radiation sciences and medical radiology. *Radiother Oncol* 1983; 1:1–22.

20. Fowler JF: Potential for increasing the differential response between tumors and normal tissues: Can proliferation rate be used? *Int J Radiat Oncol Biol Phys* 1986; 12:641–646.
21. Fowler JF: Review: Total doses in fractionated radiotherapy—Implications of new radiobiological data. *Int J Radiat Biol* 1984; 46:103–120.
22. Fowler JF: What next in fractionated radiotherapy? *Br J Cancer [Suppl VI]* 1984; 49:285S–300S.
23. Hall EJ: *Radiobiology for the Radiobiologist*, ed 3. Philadelphia, JB Lippincott, 1988.
24. Hall E, Graves RG, Phillips TL, et al (eds): Particle accelerators in radiation therapy. *Int J Radiat Oncol Biol Phys* 1982; 8:2041–2207.
25. Kinsella T, Mitchell J, Russo A, et al: The use of halogenated thymidine analogs as clinical radiosensitizers: Rationale, current status, and future prospects—Nonhypoxic cell sensitizers. *Int J Radiat Oncol Biol Phys* 1984; 10:1399–1406.
26. Lyskin AB, Mendelsohn ML: Comparison of cell cycle in induced carcinomas and their normal counterparts. *Cancer Res* 1964; 24:1131.
27. Malaise EP, Adams GE, Dische S, et al (eds): *Chemical Modifiers of Cancer Treatment*. New York, Pergamon Press, in press.
28. Malaise EP, Fertil B, Deschavanne PJ, et al: Initial slope of radiation survival curves is characteristic of the origin of primary and established cultures of human tumor cells in fibroblasts. *Radiat Res* 1987; 111:319–334.
29. Mendelsohn ML: The growth fraction: A new concept applied to tumors. *Science* 1960; 132:1496.
30. Mitchell J, Russo A, Kinsella T, et al: The use of nonhypoxic cell sensitizers in radiobiology and radiotherapy. *Int J Radiat Oncol Biol Phys* 1986; 12:1513–1518.
31. Overgaard J: Historical perspectives of hyperthermia, in Overgaard J (ed): *Introduction to Hyperthermic Oncology*, vol 2. New York, Taylor & Francis, 1984.
32. Palcic B, Skarsgard LD: Reduced oxygen enhancement ratio at low doses of ionizing radiation. *Radiat Res* 1984; 100:328–329.
33. Patt HM, Tyree EB, Straube RL, et al: Cysteine protection against x-irradiation. *Science* 1949; 110:213.
34. Peters LJ, Withers HR, Cundiff JH, et al: Radiobiological considerations in the use of total body irradiation for bone marrow transplantation. *Radiology* 1979; 131:234–247.
35. Peters LJ, Withers HR, Thames HD: Radiobiological basis for multiple daily fractionation, in Kaercher KH, Kogelnik HD, Reinartz G (eds): *Progress in Radio-Oncology*, vol 2. New York, Raven Press, 1982, pp 317–323.
36. Phillips TL, et al: Radiation protection of tumor and normal tissue by thiophosphate compounds. *Cancer* 1973; 32:528.

37. Powers WE, Tolmach LJ: A multi-component x-ray survival curve for mouse lymphosarcoma cells irradiated in vivo. *Nature* 1963; 197:710–711.

38. Raju MR, Richmond C: Physical and radiobiological aspects of negative pions with reference to radiotherapy. *Gann Monograph 9*, 1970, pp 105–121.

39. Rich TA: Intraoperative Radiotherapy: A review. *Radiother Oncol* 1986; 6:207–221.

40. Rubin P: Principles of radiation oncology and cancer radiotherapy, in Rubin P (ed): *Clinical Oncology for Medical Students and Physicians: A Multidisciplinary Approach*. New York, American Cancer Society, 1983.

41. Sinclair WK, Moreton RA: X-ray sensitivity during the cell generation cycle of cultured Chinese hamster cells. *Radiat Res* 1966; 29:450.

42. Steel GG: Cell loss as a factor in the growth rate of human tumors. *Eur J Cancer* 1967; 3:381–387.

43. Steel GG, Lamerton LF: The growth rate of human tumors. *Br J Cancer* 1966; 20:74.

44. Strandqvist M: Studien uber die kumulative Wirkung der Rontgenstrahlen bei Fraktionierung. *Acta Radiol [Suppl]* 1944; 55:1.

45. Tannock IF: The relation between cell proliferation in the vascular system and the transplanted mouse mammary tumor. *Br J Cancer* 1968; 22:258.

46. Terasima T, Tolmach LJ: Variations in several responses of HeLa cells to x-irradiation during division cycle. *Biophys J* 1965; 3:11.

47. Thames HD, Hendry JH: *Fractionation in Radiotherapy*. London, Taylor & Francis, 1987.

48. Thames HD, Peters LJ, Ang KK: Time dose considerations for normal tissue tolerance, in *Frontiers of Radiation Therapy and Oncology, Radiation Effect and Tolerance, Normal Tissue in the Optimal Treatment of Cancer*, Vaeth JM (ed), New York, S Karger, 1988, in press.

49. Thames HD, Peters LJ, Withers HR, et al: Accelerated fractionation vs hyperfractionation: Rationale for several treatments per day. *Int J Radiat Oncol Biol Phys* 1983; 9:127–138.

50. Thames HD, Withers HR, Peters LJ, et al: Changes in early and late radiation responses with altered dose fractionation. Implications for dose survival relationships. *Int J Radiat Oncol Biol Phys* 1982; 8:219–226.

51. Thomlinson RH: Effect of fractionated irradiation on the proportion of anoxic cells in an intact experimental tumor. *Br J Radiol* 1966; 39:158.

52. Thomlinson RH, Gray LH: The histological structure of some human lung cancers and the possible implications for radiotherapy. *Br J Cancer* 1955; 9:539.

53. Travis EL, Thames HD, Tucker SL, et al: Protection of mouse jejunal crypt cells by WR-2721 after fractionated doses of radiation. *Int J Radiat Oncol Biol Phys* 1986; 12:807–814.

54. Tubiana M, et al: The application of radiobiologic knowledge and cellular kinetics to radiation therapy. *Am J Roentgenol Radium Ther Nucl Med* 1968; 102:822.
55. Van Putten LM, Kahlman LF: Oxygenation status of the transplantable tumor during fractionated radiotherapy. *J Natl Cancer Inst* 1968; 40:441.
56. Williams MV, Denekamp J, Fowler JF: A review of α/β ratios for experimental tumors; Implications for clinical studies of altered fractionation. *Int J Radiat Oncol Biol Phys* 1985; 11:87–96.
57. Withers HR: Cell cycle redistribution as a factor in multi-fraction irradiation. *Radiology* 1975; 114:199–202.
58. Withers HR: The 4R's of radiotherapy, in *Advances in Radiation Biology*, vol 5. San Francisco, Academic Press, 1975.
59. Withers HR, Peters LJ: Basic principles of radiotherapy, in *Textbook of Radiotherapy*, ed 2. Philadelphia, Lea & Febiger, 1980.
60. Withers HR, Thames HD, Peters LJ: Biological basis for high RBE values for late effects of neutron irradiation. *Int J Radiat Oncol Biol Phys* 1982; 8:2071–2076.
61. Withers HR, Thames HD, Peters LJ, et al: Normal tissue radioresistance in clinical radiotherapy, in Fletcher GH, Nervi C, Withers HR (eds): *Biological Basis and Clinical Implications of Tumor Radioresistance*. New York: Masson, 1983; pp 139–152.
62. Yuhas JM: Active vs passive absorption kinetics as the basis for selective protection of normal tissues by s-2(3 amino-propylamino) ethyl-phosphorothiic-acid. *Cancer Res* 1980; 40:1519–1524.
63. Yuhas JM, Spellman JM, Culo F: The role of WR-2721 in radiotherapy and/or chemotherapy, in Brady L (ed), *Radiation Protectors*, New York, Masson, 1980, pp 303–308.
64. Yuhas JM, Storer JB: Differential chemoprotection of normal and malignant tissues. *J Natl Cancer Inst* 1969; 42:331.

Glossary

Aberration.   Atypical development or growth.

Absolute Risk Model.   Model for radiation-induced cancer in which the risk of excess cancer induced by radiation is in addition to the natural incidence. Examples are leukemia and bone cancers from ingested radionuclides.

Absorbed Dose.   Energy imparted to matter by ionizing radiation per unit mass of irradiated material. In SI units the unit of absorbed dose is the Gy which is equal to 1 J/kg.

Accelerated Fractionation.   In radiotherapy, a reduction in overall time without a change in dose per fraction or total dose.

Acentric.   Without a center; in genetics, denoting a chromosome fragment without a centromere.

Actinomycin D.   An antitumor antibiotic that appears to be a radiosensitizer; has been used alone and in combination with radiation for the treatment of cancer.

Acutely Responding Normal Tissue.   Tissues which express their injury within a few months after irradiation and are characterized by a high α/β ratio. Examples are jejunum, skin, and oral mucosa.

Adenine.   One of the two purines found in both RNA and DNA.

Albumin.   Egg white—a well-known protein.

Alopecia.   Loss of hair.

Alpha Particle (α-Particle).   A positively charged nuclear particle consisting of two protons and two neutrons, with a mass of 4 and a charge of + 2; identical to the nucleus of a helium atom. Its physical properties render it highly ionizing; therefore it is considered a high-LET radiation.

α/β Ratio. In the linear quadratic model of cell survival, the ratio of the parameters α and β that describes the shape of the survival curve or the isoeffect plot. High α/β ratios indicate little curvature in the survival curve and are typical of acutely responding normal tissues. Low α/β ratios indicate a "curvier" survival curve and are characteristic of late responding normal tissues.

"ALARA". As Low As Reasonably Achievable; guideline to be used for exposure to radiation of personnel in the radiation industries.

Amino Acid. Building block of protein; an organic acid linked by peptide bonds to form a protein.

Anabolism. Building up or synthesis of an organic compound.

Anaphase. Stage of mitosis or meiosis in which the chromosomes move from the equatorial plate toward the poles of the cell.

Anemia. Condition in which the blood is deficient in red cells, hemoglobin, or total volume; usually manifested by pallor of the skin, lack of energy, shortness of breath, and fatigability.

Angiography. Radiography of vessels following the injection of a radiopaque material into an artery, e.g., the carotid.

Ankylosing Spondylitis. Condition closely related to, or a variant of, rheumatoid arthritis.

Anomaly. Deviation from the average or norm; anything unusual, irregular, or contrary to a general rule.

Anophthalmia. Absence of one or both eyes.

Anoxia. Total oxygen deficiency.

Apoptosis. Mode of cell death characterized by nuclear fragmentation, cell lysis, and phagocytosis of the chromatin bodies by neighboring cells.

Armamentarium. Equipment and methods used in a particular field, often applied to medicine.

Arteriography. Visualization of an artery or arteries by x-rays after injection of a radiopaque contrast medium.

Ascites. Accumulation of serous fluid in the abdomen.

Asynchronous. Not occurring simultaneously.

Atrophy.   Indicates decrease in size of cells in an organ, possibly producing a decrease in size of organ.

Basal Layer.   Immature, dividing layer of cells at the base of the epidermis.

BEIR.   Biological Effects of Ionizing Radiations; advisory committee that published a report on the effects of ionizing radiation on biologic systems.

Beta Particle.   Electron (β^-) or positron (β^+) ejected from the nucleus of an atom during radioactive decay has mass identical to an electron and a charge of -1 or $+1$, respectively. β-particles from ^{32}P are used in the treatment of polycythemia vera.

Biologic Half-Life.   Time taken for one half of an administered radioactive substance to be lost through the biologic process of elimination.

Bleomycin.   Antitumor antibiotic that localizes in squamous epithelium and is presently being used in the treatment of many types of cancer—e.g., squamous carcinoma, melanoma, and Hodgkin's disease—either alone or in combination with another form of treatment; appears to potentiate the effect of radiation.

Blood Platelet.   Irregularly shaped disk, about one third to one half the size of an erythrocyte, containing no hemoglobin; necessary for blood clotting.

Bolus.   Tissue-equivalent material placed on the surface of the body to minimize the effects of an irregular surface; used in external beam radiation therapy to assure more uniform dose distribution.

Bone Marrow.   Tissue filling the cavities of bones and having a stroma of reticular fibers and cells; it may be yellow because the meshes of the reticular network are filled with fat or red because the meshes contain the precursors to the mature circulating blood cells.

Brachytherapy.   "Short distance" radiotherapy, using sealed sources; intracavitary radium for cervical carcinoma.

Californium 252.   Mixed neutron and γ-emitter; sealed sources are used in brachytherapy.

Cancer.   General, laymen's term frequently used to indicate any of the various types of malignant neoplasms.

Cancer Cord.   Named for a distinct architectural pattern observed in a human bronchial carcinoma, consisting of a central region of necrosis surrounded by a rim of viable cells.

Capillary.   Any of the smallest vessels of the blood-vascular system connecting arterioles with venules and forming networks throughout the body.

Carbogen.   95% O_2 and 5% CO_2; breathing the mixture may increase oxygen concentration in a tumor; CO_2, a vasodilator, assists in increasing the available oxygen to the tumor.

Carbohydrate.   Organic compound composed of carbon, hydrogen, and oxygen, and the primary source of energy to the cell.

Carcinogenesis.   Origin or production of all malignant neoplasms.

Carcinoma.   Malignant tumor arising from any epithelium in the body, e.g., carcinoma of the cervix, carcinoma of the larynx, and carcinoma of the skin.

Cardiac Catheterization.   Passage of a catheter (a hollow cylinder of silver, rubber, or other material) into the heart.

Cardiovascular.   Relating to the heart, blood vessels, or circulation.

Catabolism.   Breaking down of organic compounds to provide energy and other requirements for life.

Catalyst.   A substance that increases the rate of chemical reaction.

Cataract.   A clouding of the lens of the eye or its capsule, obstructing the passage of light and causing visual impairment; an opacity of the lens of the eye.

Cell.   Smallest unit of protoplasm capable of independent existence.

Centrifugation.   Process by which particles in suspension in a fluid may be separated; this is accomplished by whirling a vessel containing the fluid about in a circle; the centrifugal force throws the particles to the peripheral part of the rotating vessel.

Centrioles.   Structures of the cell to which the spindle fibers are attached during cell division.

Centromere.   Clear region of the chromosome that is necessary to the movement of the chromosome during cell division.

Cervix.   Neck or any necklike structure, especially the neck of the uterus that connects the vagina with the uterine cavity; also used in reference to structures in the neck region of the body, e.g., cervical spine or cervical lymph nodes.

Chemotherapy.   Treatment of disease by means of chemical substances or drugs.

Chondroblast.   Cell of growing cartilage tissue that is rapidly dividing and undifferentiated; intermediate in radiosensitivity.

Chondrocyte.   Nondividing, differentiated mature cartilage cell; highly radioresistant.

Chromatid.   Each of two strands formed by duplication of a chromosome that becomes visible during prophase of mitosis or meiosis.

Chromatid Aberration.   Any deviation from the normal structure of chromatids produced when irradiation occurs *after* DNA synthesis, affecting only one chromatid of a pair.

Chromosome.   Unit of genetic material responsible for directing cytoplasmic activity and transmitting hereditary information in cells.

Chromosome Aberration.   Any deviation from the normal structure of chromosomes produced when irradiation occurs *prior* to DNA synthesis; both chromatids exhibit the change in structure.

Chromosome Ring.   A chromosome with ends joined to form a circular structure.

Cirrhosis.   Fibrosis, especially of the liver, with hardening caused by excessive formation of connective tissue followed by contraction.

Clonogen.   A cell that is capable of unlimited proliferation producing a clone of genetically identical daughters; an abbreviation for clonogenic cells.

CNS (Central Nervous System).   The brain and spinal cord.

Cobalt 60.   Heavy radioactive isotope of cobalt of mass number 60 with a half-life of 5.3 years; emits β-particles and γ-rays; used in teletherapy and brachytherapy.

Code (Genetic).   System whereby particular combinations of three adjacent nucleotides in a DNA molecule control the insertion of specific amino acids in a protein molecule.

Collimator.   Device of high-absorption-coefficient material used in diagnostic and therapy units to confine an x-ray beam to a given area; in nuclear medicine, it restricts the detection of emitted radiations to those from a given area of interest.

Committed Dose Equivalent.   Dose equivalent accumulated in 50 years after intake of a radionuclide.

Congenital.   Existing at or dating from birth; acquired during in utero development and not through heredity.

Cristae.   Shelflike structures inside the mitochondria; sites of specific enzymes necessary for the production of energy.

Critical Organ.   The dose-limiting factor in a radiopharmaceutical procedure; that organ which, although it may not accumulate the greatest percentage of a radiopharmaceutical, dictates the amount of a radiopharmaceutical that can be administered.

Curie.   Unit of radioactivity in which the number of disintegrations per second equals 3.74×10^{10}; abbreviated Ci.

Cysteamine.   Radioprotectant amino acid containing a sulfhydryl group.

Cystine.   Amino acid found in most proteins; contains a sulfhydryl group; an effective radioprotectant.

Cytokinesis.   Division of the cytoplasm during telophase of mitosis or meiosis.

Cytoplasm.   Protoplasm outside the nucleus; the site of all metabolic functions in the cell.

Cytosine.   One of two pyrimidines found in both RNA and DNA.

Dermis.   Sensitive vascular layer of the skin beneath the epidermis.

Desquamation.   Denudation or peeling of the skin surface.

Dicentric.   Chromosome having two centromeres.

Differentiating Intermitotic Cells (DIM).   Cells produced by division of VIM (vegetative intermitotic cells), although actively mitotic, are more differentiated than VIM; DIM cells are less sensitive (or more resistant) to radiation than are VIM cells, e.g., intermediate and Type B spermatogonia.

Differentiation.   Sum of the processes whereby undifferentiated cells become specialized functionally and/or morphologically (structurally).

DIM. Differentiating intermitotic cells.

Diploid. Having the basic chromosome number is doubled, as in somatic cells (2n).

Direct Action. Interaction and absorption of an ionizing particle by a biologic macromolecule such as DNA, RNA, protein, or enzyme in the cell.

Disaccharide. Carbohydrate formed from two monosaccharides, e.g., table sugar.

Division Delay. Synonym for mitotic delay.

DNA (Deoxyribonucleic Acid). Double-stranded, helical structure in nucleus that contains the genetic material of the cell; composed of nitrogenous bases, 5-carbon sugars, and phosphoric acid.

DNA Synthesis. Process that doubles the amount of original DNA in such a manner that the newly formed DNA is identical to the original molecule.

D_0. An expression of radiosensitivity; graphically derived from the exponential portion of the cell survival curve.

Dose Equivalent. A quantity used for radiation protection that expresses on a common scale for all radiations, the radiation incurred by exposed persons. It is defined as the product of the absorbed dose and the quality factor. The SI unit of dose equivalent is seivert (Sv).

Dose-Modifying Compounds. Radioprotectant compounds that act by reducing the effective dose of radiation to cells.

Dose Rate. Rate at which radiation is delivered.

Dosimetry. The concept and measurement of quantity of radiation, either emitted by various sources or absorbed by body tissues.

Doubling Dose. Unit of measurement for determination of radiation effects on mutation frequency; defined as that dose of radiation which ultimately doubles the number of spontaneous mutations that arise in one generation, generally 0.5 Gy in humans.

Doubling Time. The time in which a tumor doubles in volume.

D_q. Quasi-threshold dose, the width of the shoulder region of a cell survival curve.

DRF. Dose reduction factor; the ratio of the radiation dose necessary to produce a given effect in the presence of a protecting compound to the radiation dose necessary to produce the same effect in the absence of the same compound.

Edema. Abnormal accumulation of serous fluid in connective tissue or in a serous cavity.

Effective Dose Equivalent. The sum for a specified tissue of the product of the dose equivalent in the tissue and the weighting factor for that tissue.

EKG (Electrocardiogram). Graphic record of the heart's action.

Elective Booking. A procedure used in diagnostic radiology and nuclear medicine to identify the potentially pregnant patient.

Electromagnetic Radiation. Radiation having no mass or charge, often spoken of in terms of photon or quantum (small packet of energy), e.g., radio waves, visible light, x-rays, and γ-rays.

Elkind Repair. Recovery of the shoulder on a radiation survival curve when two doses of radiation are split by several hours.

Embryo. In humans, the developing organism from conception to the end of the 6th week of gestation.

Enzyme. A protein that acts as a catalyst, inducing chemical changes in other substances, itself remaining apparently unchanged in the process.

Epidemiology. Science that deals with the incidence, distribution, and control of disease in a population.

Epidermis. Outer nonsensitive and nonvascular layer of the skin overlying the dermis.

Epilation. Hair loss; synonym for alopecia.

Equatorial Plate. Imaginary line in the center of the cell equidistant from both poles along which the chromosomes align during metaphase of mitosis and meiosis.

ER (Endoplasmic Reticulum). Double-membraned cell organelle composed of an irregular network of branching and connecting tubules, which functions in the synthesis of proteins and other substances.

Ergastoplasm. Synonym for endoplasmic reticulum.

Erythema.   Redness of the skin.

Erythroblast.   The first specifically identifiable precursor cell in red blood cell formation; located in red bone marrow.

Erythrocyte.   Red blood cell; highly radioresistant.

Esophagitis.   Inflammation of the mucous membranes of the esophagus.

Etiology.   Cause or origin of a disease or abnormal condition.

Exencephaly.   Condition in which the skull is defective, the brain being exposed or extruding; brain hernia.

External Beam Therapy.   See Teletherapy.

Fetus.   In humans, the unborn developing human from 6 weeks postconception to birth.

Fibroblasts.   Elongated cells that constitute connective tissue; of intermediate radiosensitivity.

Fibrocyte.   Cells of mature connective tissue; relatively radioresistant.

Fibrosis.   Formation of fibrous tissue, usually as a reparative or reactive process.

5 BUDR.   5-Bromodeoxyuridine; a halogenated pyrimidine; a true radiosensitizing drug.

5 FU.   5-Fluorouracil; a halogenated pyrimidine; not a true radiosensitizing drug.

5 IUDR.   5-Iododeoxyuridine; a true radiosensitizing drug.

Fixed Postmitotic Cells.   Cells that do not divide and are highly differentiated both morphologically and functionally; most radioresistant of all cells.

Fluoroscope.   Apparatus for visualizing the shadows of x-rays, which, after passing through the body, are projected onto a fluorescent screen.

FPM.   Fixed postmitotic cells.

Fractionation.   Extention of the total radiation dose in radiation therapy over a period of time, ordinarily days or weeks, in order to minimize untoward radiation effects on normal contiguous tissue.

Free Radical.   A radical in its (usually transient) uncombined state; atom or atom group carrying an unpaired electron and no charge; atom containing a single unpaired electron, rendering it highly reactive.

Gamete.   Germ cells in sexually reproducing plants and animals; in females, the oocytes, and in males, the spermatozoa.

γ-Rays.   Electromagnetic radiations originating from atomic nuclei, produced when an unstable atomic nucleus releases energy to gain stability.

Gastrointestinal.   Relating to both stomach and intestine.

Gene.   Located on a chromosome; the unit of genetic material that is responsible for directing cytoplasmic activity and transmitting hereditary information in the cell.

Germ Cell.   Cells in sexually reproducing plants and animals with a haploid number of chromosomes.

Gestation.   The carrying of the young in the uterus; pregnancy.

Gonad.   An organ that produces sex cells; the testis of a male or the ovary of a female.

G_1–Gap 1.   Period between telophase and the beginning of DNA synthesis when DNA is not replicating.

G_2–Gap 2.   Period following DNA replication and prior to mitosis.

Granulocyte.   Mature leukocyte containing cytoplasmic granules.

Growth Fraction.   The fraction of the total tumor cell population that is dividing, responsible for tumor growth.

GSD (Genetic Significant Dose).   An average figure calculated from the actual gonadal doses received by the exposed population; evaluates the genetic impact of medical/dental x-ray doses on the whole population.

Guanine.   One of two purine bases found in both DNA and RNA.

Gy.   Grey; SI unit of absorbed dose; 1 Gy = 1 J/kg = 100 rad.

Halogenated Pyrimidines.   Chemical compounds that can replace the base thymine on DNA; effective radiosensitizers, including 5-bromodeoxyuridine (5-BUDR) and 5-iododeoxyuridine (5-IUDR).

HeLa Cells.   Cells originally derived from a human carcinoma of the cervix; now grown in tissue culture.

Helix.   A spiraled structure.

Hemoglobin.   The red protein of erythrocytes that carries O_2.

Hemopoietic System.   System that deals with the formation of blood cells; includes the bone marrow, circulating blood, lymph nodes, spleen, and thymus.

Hemorrhage.   Bleeding; a flow of blood, especially if profuse.

Hepatic.   Relating to the liver.

Hepatitis.   Inflammation of the liver.

Hodgkin's Disease.   Malignant disease of the lymph nodes, characterized by enlargement of the nodes, often cervical in onset and then generalized, sometimes with enlargement of the spleen and liver.

Homologous.   Having the same relative position, value, or structure; applied to chromosomes; two chromosomes with identical sequence and type of genes.

Hydrocephaly.   Water on the brain.

Hydroxyurea (HU).   Drug that synchronizes a population of cells; sometimes used in combination with radiation therapy.

Hyperbaric Oxygen (HPO).   Pure O_2 at 3 atm pressure, tried in radiation therapy to increase available O_2 to tumor cells and overcome the oxygen effect.

Hyperfractionation.   In radiotherapy, an increase in the number of fractions and reduction in dose per fraction in the same overall time.

Hyperthyroidism.   Excessive functional activity of the thyroid gland resulting in a condition marked by increased metabolic rate and enlargement of the thyroid gland.

Hypoplasia.   Loss of cells, loss of tissue, or organ atrophy due to destruction of some of the elements and not merely to their general reduction in size.

Hypoxia.   Decreased amount of oxygen; oxygen deficiency, less than physiologically normal amount.

Hypoxic Cell Sensitizers.   Drugs that selectively sensitize hypoxic cells; one example is the nitrofurans, such as NDPP-p-nitro, 3-dimethylaminopropiophenone hydrochloride.

Immune System.   Cells (lymphocytes and other white cells) and organs (spleen, lymph nodes, and thymus) that provide natural defense against disease.

Immunotherapy.   Treatment directed at the immune system.

In Utero.   Within the womb; not yet born.

In Vitro.   In glassware or in an artificial environment, outside the living body; opposite of in vivo (in a living system).

In Vivo.   In the living body; referring to vital chemical and other processes as distinguished from those occurring in the test tube (in vitro).

Indirect Action.   Absorption of ionizing radiation by the medium in which cell organelles are suspended, primarily water.

Inflammation.   Local response to cellular injury marked by capillary dilation, leukocytic infiltration, redness, heat, pain, and swelling; serves as a mechanism initiating the elimination of toxic agents and of damaged tissue.

Inorganic.   Not organic; not relating to living organisms; in chemistry, referring to compounds not containing carbon, e.g., mineral salts (Na + K).

Insulin.   A well-known protein (polypeptide) produced by the pancreas involved in the regulation of metabolism, especially carbohydrate metabolism.

Integral Dose.   Incorporates volume, in grams, of tissue irradiated; defined as gram-rads.

Interphase.   The nondividing or intermitotic period between two successive divisions of a cell.

Interphase Death.   Cell death before entering mitosis.

Interstitial Therapy.   Placement of sealed radioactive sources directly in a malignant tumor.

Intracavitary Therapy.   Placement of sealed radioactive sources within a body cavity close to the tumor; the sources are held in place by applicators, e.g., in the treatment of carcinoma of the cervix.

Inversions.   A turning inward, upside down, or in any direction contrary to the existing one; a type of chromosome aberration.

Ion.   An atom or group of atoms that carries a positive or negative charge as a result of having lost or gained one or more electrons.

Irradiation.   Subjection to radiation.

Isoeffect Curve.   Similar curve, a line formed from plotting total dose and overall treatment time on a double logarithmic plot; relates treatment schedule to clinical results.

Isoeffect Plot.   Dose for equal effect, e.g., LD_{50} plotted against dose per fraction or dose rate.

keV/μm.   The unit of expression for LET equal to the energy deposited per unit distance of path traveled by a charged particle.

Late Responding Normal Tissue.   Tissues that express their injury months after radiation and are characterized by small α/β ratios. Examples are kidney, lung, and spinal cord.

Latent Period.   The time between injury and the expression of that injury by a cell or tissue.

Law of Ancel and Vitemberger.   Inherent susceptibility of any cell to damage by ionizing radiation is the same, but the time of appearance of radiation-induced damage differs among different types of cells. Named after the two investigators responsible for this determination.

Law of Bergonié and Tribondeau.   Ionizing radiation is more effective against cells that are actively mitotic, undifferentiated, and have a long dividing future; named after the two investigators who determined this effect; considered a byword in radiobiology.

LD_{50}.   Dose to produce lethality in 50% of the subjects by a given time, e.g., $LD_{50/30}$, in 30 days.

Lieberkühn, Crypts of.   Named after the German anatomist. Nests of cells at the base of the villi in the intestine; a rapidly dividing undifferentiated stem cell population; relatively radiosensitive.

Lesion.   Abnormal change in structure of an organ or part due to injury or disease.

LET.   Linear energy transfer.

Leukemia.   An acute or chronic disease of unknown cause in humans and other warm-blooded animals characterized by an abnormal increase in the number of leukocytes (white blood cells) in tissue and blood.

Leukemogenic.   Leukemia-causing.

Leukocyte.   Any of the white or colorless nucleated cells that occur in blood.

Leukopenia. Pronounced reduction in the number of white blood cells in the circulating blood.

Linear Accelerator. Device in which electrons are accelerated striking a target or window, generating x-rays of greater than 4 mV; teletherapy unit used in radiation therapy.

Linear Energy Transfer. Rate at which energy is deposited as a charged particle travels through matter.

Linear Quadratic (LQ) Model. Model in which the survival rate is a linear and quadratic function of dose: $E = \alpha D + \beta D^2$.

Lipid. Class of organic compounds that, with proteins and carbohydrates, constitutes the principal structural components of living cells. Functions include energy storage, protection of the body against cold, and assistance in digestive processes.

Lumbar. Relating to the loins; the part of the back and sides between the ribs and the pelvis.

Lymphocytes. White blood cells formed in lymphoid tissue throughout the body, e.g., lymph nodes, spleen, thymus, tonsils, Peyer's patches, and sometimes bone marrow; highly radiosensitive.

Lymphoid. Resembling lymph (a pale coagulable fluid that consists of a liquid portion resembling blood plasma containing white blood cells).

Lymphoma. A general term that includes various abnormally proliferative neoplastic diseases of the lymphoid tissues, e.g., lymphosarcoma and Hodgkin's disease; ordinarily termed malignant lymphoma.

Lyse. To break up or disintegrate, often applied to cells.

Lysosome. A single-membraned cell organelle that contains enzymes capable of breaking down proteins, DNA, and some carbohydrates.

Macromolecule. A polymer, notably proteins, nucleic acids, and polysaccharides.

Malignant. Resistant to treatment, occurring in severe form and frequently fatal; tending to become worse; in the case of a neoplasm, having properties of invasion, metastasis, and uncontrollable growth.

Mammal. Any of a class (mammalia) of higher vertebrates comprising humans and all other animals that nourish their young with milk secreted by mammary glands and have skin usually more or less covered with hair.

Mastectomy. Amputation of the breast.

Matrix. The ground cytoplasm, or medium, in which the cell organelles are suspended.

Maturation Depletion. Process of depletion of mature sperm by depopulation of spermatogonia.

Maximum Permissible Dose. The allowable radiation dose at which there is assumed to be relatively small biologic risk to occupationally exposed persons and to the general population; the present MPD for total body exposure of occupationally exposed persons is 5 rem/year after age 18.

Megakaryocytes. Precursor cells for blood platelets; the least radiosensitive of bone marrow stem cells.

Meiosis. Process of cell division in germ cells, consisting of two cellular divisions but only one DNA replication, resulting in formation of four gametocytes, each containing half the number of chromosomes found in somatic cells.

Melanoma. Malignant neoplasm derived from cells that are capable of forming melanin.

Meson. An unstable nuclear particle, first observed in cosmic rays, with a mass between that of the electron and the proton; can be either charged or neutral; investigational radiation therapy modality.

Metabolism. The sum of the processes in the building up (anabolism) and destruction (catabolism) of protoplasm incidental to the cell life.

Metaphase. Stage of mitosis or meiosis in which the chromosomes become aligned on the equatorial plate of the cell with the centromeres mutually repelling each other.

Metastasis. The appearance of neoplasms in parts of the body remote from the site of the primary tumor.

Methotrexate (MTX). A drug used to synchronize a population of cells, sometimes used in combination with radiation therapy.

Microcephaly. Abnormal smallness of the head (brain).

Microcurie. One millionth of a curie; 3.7×10^4 disintegrations per second; abbreviated μCi.

Microphthalmia. Small size of one or both eyeballs.

Millicurie. One thousandth of a curie; 3.7×10^7 disintegrations per second; abbreviated mCi.

Mitochondria. Organelles of the cell cytoplasm consisting of two sets of membranes, a smooth continuous outer coat and a convoluted inner membrane arranged in folds, that form shaftlike structures called cristae; the powerhouses of the cell, producing energy for cellular functions.

Mitosis. Process of cellular reproduction in somatic cells whereby one parent cell divides to form two daughter cells with the same chromosome number and DNA content as the original parent cell; consists of four phases—prophase, metaphase, anaphase, and telophase.

Mitotic Delay. A cellular response to irradiation; cells are delayed from entering mitosis for a varying period of time, depending on dose.

Mitotic Index. Ratio of the number of cells in mitosis at any one time to the total number of cells in the population.

Molecule. The smallest possible quantity of a substance, composed of two or more similar or dissimilar atoms that exists independently and still retains the chemical properties of the substance of which it forms a part, e.g., O_2, H_2O, and H_2.

Mongoloid. Child born with a congenital idiocy of unknown cause having slanting eyes, a broad short skull, and broad hands with short fingers.

Monomer. Simple molecular units that are individually stable and have specific chemical characteristics and properties.

Monosaccharide. A carbohydrate not decomposable to simple sugars, e.g., glucose and fructose.

Morphology. Study of the structure or form of biologic materials.

MPD. See Maximum Permissible Dose.

Mucositis. Inflammation of the mucous membranes of the oral cavity.

Multidisciplinary Approach.   A combination of cancer treatment modalities, e.g., radiation therapy, surgery, chemotherapy, and immunotherapy.

Multipotential Connective Tissue Cells.   Cells that divide irregularly and are more differentiated than either VIM (vegetative intermitotic cells) or DIM (differentiating intermitotic cells); intermediate radiosensitivity, e.g., endothelial cells.

Multitarget Model.   Assumes the presence of many cells, all of which must be inactivated for death to occur.

Mutagen.   Any agent that causes the production of a mutation, e.g., virus, drugs, and radiation.

Mutation.   Alteration in the sequence of base pairs on the DNA molecule or in the amount or volume of DNA.

Mutation Frequency.   The number of spontaneous or induced mutations that arise per generation.

Myelitis.   Inflammation of the spinal cord.

Myelocytes.   Precursor cells in the bone marrow to circulating white cells; relatively radiosensitive.

Myeloid.   (1) Of or relating to the spinal cord. (2) Of, relating to, or resembling bone marrow.

n (Extrapolation Number).   One of three graphic parameters used to define the cell survival curve; determined by extrapolating the exponential portion of the cell survival curve to its intersection with the Y axis.

n (Haploid Number).   Refers to the number of chromosomes in germ cells.

NCRP.   National Commission on Radiation Protection and Measurement.

Necrosis.   The pathologic death of one or more cells or of a portion of tissue or organ, resulting from irreversible damage.

Neonatal.   Relating to the period immediately succeeding birth and continuing through the first month of life.

Neoplasm.   A new growth, e.g., a tumor, not necessarily malignant.

Nephritis.   Acute or chronic inflammation of the kidneys.

Neuroblast.   An embryonic nerve cell.

Neutron.   An uncharged particle in the nucleus of an atom.

Nominal Standard Dose (NSD).   A unit incorporating total tumor dose, number of fractions, and overall treatment time, expressed in the formula: $D = (NSD)T^{0.11}N^{0.24}$, where D = total dose, N = number of fractions, and T = overall treatment time.

Nondivision Death.   See Interphase Death.

Nonmitotic Death.   See Interphase Death.

Nonstochastic Effects.   Effect for which severity increases with dose and for which a threshold usually exists, e.g., death after irradiation of an organ or of the total body.

NSD.   See Nominal Standard Dose.

Nuclear Medicine.   The clinical field of study concerned with the diagnostic and therapeutic use of radionuclides, excluding the therapeutic use of sealed radiation sources.

Nucleic Acid.   Major class of organic compounds in the cell composed of a sugar or derivative of a sugar, phosphoric acid, and a base; RNA and DNA.

Nucleolus.   Mass of stainable material in the cell nucleus that houses nuclear RNA.

Nucleotide.   The three components of DNA taken together, including a nitrogenous base, a 5-carbon sugar, and phosphoric acid.

Nucleus.   Center; applied to cells, a portion of protoplasm containing the genetic material, separated from the cytoplasm by a membrane.

Occlude.   To close or bring together.

OER (Oxygen Enhancement Ratio).   Ratio of dose required to produce a given biologic response in the absence of oxygen to the dose required to produce the same response in the presence of oxygen.

Oncogene.   Genes whose expression appears to be linked to conversion of normal cells to cancer cells.

Oocyte.   The immature ovum.

Organ.   A differentiated structure consisting of cells and tissues and performing some specific function, such as respiration, secretion, or digestion.

Organelle. Specialized structures in a cell performing specific functions.

Organic. Of, relating to, or containing carbon compounds.

Organogenesis. Formation of organs during development; in humans, the period from the 2nd to 6th week postconception.

Orthovoltage. Medium voltage of 250 kV, referred to in radiation therapy as deep therapy.

Osmotic Pressure. The force under which a solvent moves from a solution of lower solute concentration to a solution of higher solute concentration when these solutions are separated by a selectively permeable membrane.

Osteoblast. Bone-forming cells; moderately radiosensitive.

Osteoclast. Bone-resorbing cells; moderately radiosensitive.

Osteosarcoma. Malignant neoplasm of bone.

Ovarian Follicle. One of the saclike enclosures in the ovary containing an ovum.

Overshoot, Mitotic. Increased number of cells in mitosis.

Oxygen Effect. Specific name given to the response of cells to radiation in the presence of oxygen.

Oxygen Enhancement Ratio. See OER.

Oxygen Tension. Pressure excreted by oxygen proportional to the percentage of oxygen molecules present in the total volume of blood.

Palliative. Relieving; causing to reduce in severity; often used in relation to a method of treatment of a disease.

Pancarditis. Inflammation of all the structures of the heart, including endocardium, myocardium, and epicardium.

Pancreas. A large compound gland of vertebrates that secretes digestive enzymes and the hormone insulin.

Pancytopenia. Pronounced reduction in the number of erythrocytes, all types of white blood cells, and blood platelets in the circulating blood.

Papain. Proteolytic enzyme used as a protein digestant and meat tenderizer.

Parenchyma.   The distinguishing or specific cells of a gland or organ, contained in and supported by the connective tissue framework or stroma.

Particle.   Type of ionizing radiation that has mass and charge.

Peptide Bond.   Chemical bond joining two amino acids.

Pericarditis.   Inflammation of the pericardium (the membrane covering the heart).

Petechial Hemorrhages.   Minute hemorrhagic spots, of pin point to pinhead size, in blood vessel walls.

Physical Half-Life.   Time required for one half of the atoms of a specific radionuclide to undergo disintegration.

Physiology.   Study of the normal vital processes of living animal and vegetable organisms.

Pion.   Pi-meson.

Pneumonitis.   Inflammation of the lungs.

Polycythemia Vera.   Malignant disease of red blood cells; actually an increased number of RBCs.

Polymer.   Two or more monomers joined by polymerization to form a chain consisting essentially of repeating structural units.

Polymerization.   Process by which polymers are joined.

Polysaccharide.   Carbohydrate that can be decomposed into two or more molecules of monosaccharides.

Portal.   Opening or window; in radiation therapy, that area of the body being treated.

Potentially Lethal Damage.   Damage that can be repaired between irradiation and the subsequent mitosis, and which is lethal if not repaired.

Potentiate.   To enhance; in radiation, to enhance the response of cells, tissues, organs, etc., by addition of some substance, e.g., oxygen.

Precursor.   Anything that precedes another or from which another is derived; forerunner.

Primary Repair.   Replacement of damaged cells in the organ by the same cell type present before radiation; also called *regeneration*.

Procreate.   To produce offspring; generate.

Prodromal Stage.   Initial; in radiation, that stage of response to an acute total body dose of radiation characterized by nausea, vomiting, and diarrhea (often referred to as N-V-D syndrome).

Prophase.   First stage of mitosis or meiosis consisting of linear contraction and increasing thickness of the chromosomes, accompanied by division of the centriole.

Protein.   One of the four major classes of cellular organic compounds; macromolecules consisting of long sequences of α-amino acids in peptide linkage; constitutes approximately 15% of cell content and is the most plentiful carbon-containing compound in the cell.

Protoplasm.   The colloidal complex of organic and inorganic substances and water that constitutes the living cell.

Puck, T. T., and Marcus, T. I..   Investigators who conducted a classic radiobiologic experiment and constructed the cell survival curve.

Purine.   One of two categories of nitrogenous bases found in DNA; includes the bases adenine and guanine.

Pyelogram.   Radiogram of the renal pelvis and uterer.

Pyrimidine.   One of two categories of nitrogenous bases found in DNA; includes the bases thymine and cytosine.

Quality Factor.   Factor used for radiation protection purposes that accounts for the differences in biologic effects of different kinds of radiation.

Quasi-Threshold Dose (D_q).   Defines the width of the shoulder region of the cell survival curve and is the dose at which point the curve becomes exponential.

Rad.   Old unit for absorbed dose; 1 rad is 0.01 J absorbed/kg of matter, 110 ergs/g and 0.01 Gy.

Radiation Syndrome.   A group of signs and symptoms that occur together, characterizing the system most affected by total body exposure to ionizing radiation.

Radiation Tolerance.   The limit of radiation exposure a normal tissue can receive and still remain functional.

Radical (noun).   A group of elements or atoms usually passing intact from one compound to another, but usually incapable of prolonged existence in a free state.

Radiobiology.   Study of the effects of ionizing radiation on living things.

Radionuclide.   Unstable form (or forms) of a given element, all having the same number of protons but a varying number of neutrons.

Radiopharmaceutical.   A chemical or drug to which radionuclide has been added.

Radioprotectants.   Chemicals and drugs that diminish the response of cells to radiation.

Radiosensitizers.   Chemicals and drugs that enhance radiation response of cells.

Radiotherapy.   Treatment of disease with ionizing radiation.

Radium.   Radioactive, shiny, white, metallic element that resembles barium chemically, occurs in combination in minute quantities in minerals (e.g., pitchblende), emits α-particles and γ-rays to form radon, and is used chiefly in luminous materials and in the treatment of cancer.

RBC.   Erythrocyte or red blood cell; relatively radioresistant.

RBE.   Relative biologic effect: RBE = dose in Gy from 250 keV x-ray/dose in Gy from another radiation source to produce the same biologic response

Regeneration.   Replacement of damaged cells in the organ by the same cell type present before radiation; also called primary repair.

Relative Biologic Effect.   Term relating the ability of radiations with different LET ranges to produce a specific biologic response; comparison of a dose of test radiation to a dose of 250 KeV x-ray, both producing the same biologic response.

Relative Risk Model.   Model for radiation-induced cancers in which the effect is to increase the natural incidence at all ages.

Rem.   A special unit for dose equivalent; 1 rem = 0.01 Sv.

Replication.   Repeated formation of the same molecule, as of DNA.

Reproductive Failure.   The inability of the cell to undergo repeated divisions after irradiation.

Reproductive Integrity.   Ability of cells to divide many times.

Resectable.   Amenable to surgical removal.

Resolve.   To find an answer to; to clear up.

Respiratory System. A system of organs serving the function of respiration consisting of the nose, pharynx, trachea, and lungs.

Restitution. Restoration, as in chromosome restitution.

RET (Rad Equivalent Therapy). Unit of expression of NSD.

Reverting Postmitotic Cells. Cells that do not normally undergo mitosis but retain the capability of division under specific circumstances; relatively radioresistant.

Ribonucleic Acid. One of two general types of nucleic acid that functions primarily in protein synthesis; has D-ribose as its sugar constituent and adenine, guanine, cytosine, and uracil as bases; found both in the nucleus and cytoplasm of cells.

Ribosome. A protoplasmic organelle containing ribonucleic acid; necessary for protein synthesis.

RNA. Ribonucleic acid.

RPM. See Reverting Postmitotic Cells.

S Period. Synthesis; replication; phase of cell after G_1 period and prior to G_2 period when DNA is duplicated.

Sarcoma. A malignant neoplasm arising from relatively nonrenewing tissue of mesodermal origin (as connective tissue, bone, cartilage, or striated muscle).

Sclerosis. Pathologic hardening of tissue, especially from overgrowth of fibrous tissue or increase in interstitial tissue.

Scoliosis. Lateral curvature of the spine.

Sebaceous Gland. One of a large number of glands in the dermis that usually open into the hair follicles and secrete an oily, semifluid substance.

Secondary Repair. Replacement of the original radiation damaged cells by a different cell type—usually one which forms connective tissue resulting in a scar; also called fibrosis.

Sensitivity, Conditional. Modification of cellular radiation response by external factors.

Sensitivity, Inherent. The response of the cell to radiation due to characteristics specific to the cell (mitotic activity and differentiation).

SI. International System of Units (Système International d'Unites).

Sievert. SI unit of dose equivalent. 1 Sv = 1 J/kg = 100 rem.

Skin Erythema Dose (SED). That acute dose of radiation (10 Gy) which causes skin erythema.

Somatic Cells. All cells of the body other than germ cells.

Spermatozoa. Mature, differentiated, functional cells of the testes.

Spina Bifida. Defect in the spinal column in which there is absence of the vertebral arches, and through which the spinal membranes, with or without spinal cord tissue, may protrude.

Split-Course Treatment Schedule. Administering the total therapeutic dose in two segments or courses, separated by a variable rest interval during which treatment is not given.

Split-Dose Recovery. Increase in survival when a dose is split into two equal fractions separated by various intervals of time.

Spontaneous Mutation. Naturally occurring alteration in the structure, volume, or amount of DNA.

Stem Cells. Cells capable of self renewal and differentiation to produce the various types of cells in a tissue or organ.

Stickiness, Chromosome. Clumping of chromosomes due to irradiation.

Stochastic Effects. Literally means "random in nature." Effects for which the probability of occurrence increases as a function of radiation dose. Stochastic effects generally are assumed not to exhibit a threshold.

Strandqvist, M. Did classic study in 1944 relating various fractionation schedules to the cure of skin cancer and normal tissue tolerance.

Stricture. A circumscribed narrowing or stenosis (closing) of a tubular structure, e.g., of the esophagus.

Stroma. The supporting framework, usually of connective tissue, of an organ, gland, or other structure; distinguished from the parenchyma.

Sublethal Damage. Nonlethal damage that either can be repaired or can accumulate and become lethal if further dose is given.

Sulfhydryl. Sulfur and hydrogen bound together, designated SH.

Supervoltage.   Megavoltage; greater than 1,000 V.

Synchronous.   Occurring simultaneously.

Syndrome.   A group of signs and symptoms that occur together and characterize a particular abnormality or disease.

Synthesis.   (1) Formation of compounds by the union of simpler compounds or elements. (2) A building up; a putting together.

Systemic.   Relating to a system or to the entire organism.

Systems.   Multicellular—a group of organs made up of millions of cells that together perform one or more vital functions, e.g., digestion, respiration, or circulation.

Target Cell.   A renewing cell whose death contributes to the reduction in tissue function or to tissue damage.

Target Organ.   The organ of interest in a radiopharmaceutical or radionuclide procedure.

$TD_{5/5}$.   That dose which, when given to a population of patients, results in the minimum (5%) severe complication rate within 5 years posttreatment.

$TD_{50/5}$.   That dose which, when given to a population of patients, results in the maximum (50%) severe complication rate in 5 years.

Technetium 99m. ^{99m}Tc; a metastable radionuclide formed by the decay of molybdenum; decays by gamma emission and has a half-life (physical) of 6 hours; widely used in nuclear medicine.

Telangiectasis.   Dilation of previously existing small or terminal vessels of an organ.

Teletherapy.   Radiotherapy treatment "at a distance," generally refers to treatment administered from outside the body.

Telophase.   Final stage of mitosis or meiosis, beginning when migration of chromosomes to the poles of the cell is complete.

10-Day Rule.   Rule suggested by the National Commission on Radiation Protection and Measurement recommending that all nonemergency diagnostic procedures involving the pelvis of women of childbearing age be conducted during the first 10 days of the menstrual cycle when the probability of pregnancy is very small.

Thoracic.   Relating to the thorax or chest.

Threshold. Point at which a stimulus begins to produce a sensation; lower limit of perception of a stimulus.

Thrombosis. Formation of a blood clot.

Thymine. A pyrimidine nitrogenous base of DNA only.

Tissue Culture. Growing of animal and human cells in a bottle or tube by providing nutrients.

Tolerance Dose. Concept that expresses the minimal and maximal injuries acceptable for different organs and the doses at which they occur.

Translocation. Transposition of two segments between nonhomolgous chromosomes as a result of abnormal breakage.

Transverse Myelitis. Inflammation involving the entire thickness of the spinal cord.

Trauma. An injury (as a wound) to living tissue caused by an extrinsic agent.

Treatment Field. In radiation therapy, that area of the body being treated.

2n Number (Diploid Number). The number of chromosomes in somatic cells.

250 keV X-Ray. Orthovoltage radiation.

Vasculature. Relating to or containing blood vessels.

Vegetative Intermitotic Cells. A group of rapidly dividing undifferentiated cells that have short lifetimes; most radiosensitive.

Villi. Fingerlike projections in the lining of the intestine.

VIM. See Vegetative Intermitotic Cells.

Virus. Any of a large group of submicroscopic agents consisting of nucleic acids and a protein coat that are capable of growth and multiplication only in living cells, causing various diseases.

X-Rays. Electromagnetic radiations originating from the orbital electrons of an atom.

Y-12 Accident.   Reactor accident at the Y-12 plant, Oak Ridge, Tennessee, in 1958, in which five persons were exposed to mixed neutron-gamma radiation, receiving doses estimated at 298 to 461 rem; all incurred radiation injuries but recovered.

Zygote.   Diploid cell resulting from union of a sperm and an ovum.

Index